DEDICATION

To the patients and colleagues who inspire my writing.

TABLE OF CONTENTS

Introduction 1

Bearing Witness 5

   Caring for Lucy 6

   Lies, White Lies and the Truth 12

   Shining Light in Dark Places 21

   Antibiotics, Por Favor 29

   Second Guessing the Second Opinion 37

   Field Clinics in Honduras 44

Mystery 53

   Reborn in Honduras 54

   The Pilgrim's Journey 62

   Dog Pals 70

   Meeting Daniel 75

   Denial: Titrating the Truth 79

   Expectations, Disappointments and Surprises: The Rough Waters of Narcotic Dependence 86

   Living and Dying Well 93

Wounded Healers 105

   Confessions 106

End of the Medical Deity 113

Reflections on an Untimely Death 117

The Call Came..127

On the Navajo Reservation 137

The Gesture 144

Circle Back Home...152

Epilogue 168

Discussion Questions...176

Introduction

I am a *sin eater*. Until just a century ago in Europe, a sin eater, usually a poor man, was invited to have a meal at the bedside of a dying person. A crust of bread or a cake, specially baked for the occasion, was placed on the breast of the ill individual or passed over the body. The sin eater often recited a prayer and washed the bread down with water or ale and a pinch of salt. Through this ritual, the sins of the dying were absorbed, guaranteeing the rapid passage of the dying man's soul through purgatory and on to heaven. Due to their unsavory work, sin eaters were treated as outcasts, often considered to be witches, and the Roman Catholic Church regularly excommunicated them. In Asian traditions, they took on the karma of the dying individual.

As a family physician, I am not poor and I can't imagine that I guarantee any patient's entrance into heaven. Due to the moral overtone of "sin," I'll broaden the definition to "troubles." I listen to the stories of my patients' lives -- their hardships, heartbreaks and missteps. I see the suffering of chronic pain and disabling illness, the paralysis of anxiety and the bleakness of depression. I witness the compulsions that result in addiction to cigarettes and drugs. I hear about the habits that make diabetes hard to control and keep the scale registering in the obese range. I watch each patient struggle with the hand life has dealt.

The act of listening to these troubles, sometimes confessions, is a vital part of healing, healing for patients and for me. At times I glimpse a patient's inner light, an incandescence for the briefest moment, like catching the morning sunlight angled on a spider's web bedecked with dew. I bear witness to the resourcefulness and ingenuity as well as the mire. We celebrate the joys and successes as well as problem solve the challenges. Regardless, as a healer my duty is to honor and hold the story. This in itself is healing for the patient and sometimes all I have to offer.

In the process, I become aware of my own imperfections, my impatience with some patients, my irritation at another's immobility; my own demons, bad habits and struggles. Examining these enables me to become a better healer, a better person.

We are all sinners. Today the M.D., Medical Deity is dead. Managed care, managing costs and fraud in medicine have abolished the physician's autonomy. Efforts to examine safety and quality remind everyone that physicians are human. We are not perfect; we can and do make mistakes. The professionalism curriculum, which has seen a new dawn of interest in medical schools, encourages self-evaluation and self-reflection.

In my career, I did not purchase a practice and stay to deliver the babies of the babies I also helped bring into the world. Although there is a magic and familiarity in this, the practice of medicine has changed allowing more options. I took the opportunity to practice in a community clinic, study for my Masters in Public Health, work for a health system, teach in an academic setting and see patients in a rural clinic. During vacations, between jobs and brief leaves of absence, I worked on the Navajo reservation and in international settings, primarily Central America and the former Soviet Union. In most of these settings, I have had the privilege of teaching students.

Forces in medical training often try to squeeze the humanness out of us, try to convince us that we are robots and that we must function without feeling. In emergencies, we run the risk of ignoring our own emotional responses because speed and competence, steady hands and voices are demanded. Because the buck stops with us, taking charge demands that we buckle our emotions under a tight belt. When I respond to an emergency, I must act quickly following the ABCs — airway, breathing, circulation. I've told myself many times to get a grip, that this is not the time to feel, and I summon up "Medical Mode." Mentally my pointer finger pushes the clear hold button on an old black rotary phone. My emotions and reactions are shoved away and I shift into gear — time to act *now.*

As a teacher of medical students and family physicians, I fight to help young doctors stay tuned into their feelings. Acknowledgment of our own feelings can be the key to figuring out what is going on with a patient. For example, this patient makes me exhausted, drains my energy. Is he depressed? That patient really grates on me. Why? Self-reflection often gives us clues.

After the crisis, it is essential to release the hold button and wander through the feelings. To sit with and explore my own emotional responses is painful but necessary, because buried in them are clues for my own personal growth. It may sound clichéd, but in the healing of patients, I heal myself.

During the course of this collection, you will journey with me into the urban and rural United States, as well as to international locations. In all of these places I received more than I gave. Doctoring has been a tremendous privilege these twenty-some years. I am grateful to the wise teachers I have had along the way -- other physicians, students and the patients who have either entrusted their care to me or met me on the other side of the clinic/hospital door.

All names and identifying characteristics have been altered.

Bearing Witness

The most beautiful as well as the most ugly inclinations of man are not part of a fixed biologically given human nature, but result from the social process which creates man.

Erich Fromm, U.S. (German-born) psychologist (1900 - 1980)

‡ ‡ ‡

With certain people we may get to try on a greater wholeness for a time, to actually experience being more. These experiences are a sort of grace.

Rachel Naomi Remen
Kitchen Table Wisdom, Freedom, Introduction (1996)

‡ ‡ ‡

Caring for Lucy

After two quick taps on the door, I enter the exam room. It's Saturday afternoon at the urgent care clinic. As the on-call doc, I cover twelve-hour shifts on the weekend. A young girl wearing yellow shorts and a striped top perches on a red plastic chair waiting for me; she chews on her nails. Her mother sits beside her on a too-small chair; she looks to be in her late thirties. Her dark hair is combed but greasy, and her clothes are clean but worn. She smiles when I greet them; her teeth need work.

"How can I help you?" I ask and take a seat next to them at the computer. Another hour and I can head home and get back to planting my vegetable garden.

Lucy stares at her shorts, then looks up at me through a fringe of dark bangs, her green eyes startling against her olive-tinged skin. "Sometimes I can't see," she says.

Her mother starts, "It's been going on for about a month -- feeling sick to her stomach, too. I wanted to make an appointment with her doctor, but they said she left the clinic." This helps explain why they are at urgent care, rather than the clinic that serves this city of 80,000 and the surrounding rural area. I pull up Lucy's medical record on the computer screen. She is nine years old. No labs, no past visits to guide me. My mind races ahead cataloguing the concerns of nausea and vision complaints: diabetes, brain tumor, head injury . . . what else?

I pat the exam table. "Lucy, climb up here."

Lucy does not hesitate and the exam paper crinkles as she settles in. She remains stoical while I examine her eyes and tell her to "follow the light" with the fundoscope, which she does without a problem. I draw close, the sour smell of sweat, and peer through the fundoscope to see the back of her eye (retina) and its vessels. Both sides appear normal. Then I cover one wary eye and ask her to count my fingers, she misses a few. I listen to her heart and lungs and palpate her abdomen. All fine. No bruises. I take special care with the neurologic exam. Lucy laughs when I ask her to smile, shut her eyes, and stick out her tongue. After walking heel to toe in her grubby tennis shoes, as if she were on a tight rope, she does a little twirl then sits down next to her mother. "All normal," I say and probe for more history as my attention flips between Lucy and her mother. "Do your clothes fit the same? Has anyone hurt you? Do you have a bike? Have you fallen?"

Lucy inspects her nails or fingers the hem of her shorts as she answers my questions, "Yes . . . No . . . No . . . No." Her mother catches my eye then gazes toward Lucy with concern.

"Are you afraid of anything? Anyone?" I ask.

Lucy examines her thumb and picks at the chipping pink polish. Her mother and I wait, in the silence. Then, still gazing at her lap, Lucy whispers, "Someone has a knife." I lean in to hear her. "I am afraid of the knife."

Her mother places her arm around Lucy's shoulders. "My boyfriend Tom's ex-wife lives in our complex. They have a four-year-old kid who's out of control, a biter and a kicker. The ex tells Lucy that Tom's a mean man who will hurt her."

I nod and look directly at Lucy. "Has Tom hurt you, Lucy?"

Lucy continues to stare at her lap, but shakes her head, her short hair flapping. My gut tells me that I've found the root of the problem, but I need to rule out the physical causes, which means more tests including reading the eye chart. I explain all this and ask if they have questions. "We'll talk again after you're through, okay?"

Mother nods her head. Lucy continues to scrutinize her fingernails.

I find the saviest nurse and ask her to have Lucy read the eye chart. "She may not cooperate, but see what you can find out." The nurse smiles and nods; I have an ally.

Meanwhile, I see other patients with more straightforward problems: strep throat, a urinary tract infection, a broken finger, a bruised tailbone. In between each visit, I check for Lucy's lab results. The nurse reports that Lucy intermittently recognized the letters on the eye chart, but identified the colors of the nurse's smock, the numbers on her watch, and other items on the wall without a mistake.

I face the door to Lucy's exam room, take a deep breath, tap twice and enter. Lucy's two sisters and a family friend have joined them. I sit on the stool and show Lucy and her mother the reports, explaining that the lab tests are completely normal. "I'm concerned about your worries, Lucy," I say. "They might be the cause of your symptoms." Lucy stares past me, saying nothing. I ask the family friend to take Lucy and her sisters to the waiting room so that I can talk with her mother alone. Lucy slips off her chair and out the door, trailing behind her sisters and the friend. Her mother follows them out of the room with her eyes. She continues to watch the door until I call her name.

I review Lucy's normal exam and the lab tests again and ask what her mother thinks. She picks at her cuticle, then clears her throat and murmurs, "I'm not surprised."

I consider where to start. Will mother be in denial about this boyfriend's threats? Has he hurt her? Is she able to protect her child? "You have other children," I say.

And her story begins. It is her and the three children; Lucy is the middle child. Tom does not live in the complex, but comes over frequently to visit his child who lives down the hall. "I like the manager at the complex. She's very helpful. Told me the smartest thing I did was not to let Tom move in with us. I hate to move, but I think it's the only way to make Lucy feel safe and get Tom out of our lives."

"Has Tom hurt you or the kids?" I ask.

She shakes her head emphatically and sighs. "I've been there, with Lucy's dad." I notice the worry lines in her thirty-something forehead. "I left Lucy's dad when she was just a baby. Stayed in the shelter with my two kids." She knows about orders of protection and is aware of the local domestic violence shelter. "An order of protection will piss Tom off. It'd be easier to move."

I imagine the hassle of moving three children: clothes, toys, and household items. As we talk I feel myself sink into the filaments of a spider's web. Tom has not hit her or the kids, but tells her that she spends too much money on food. "He says when we are together it'll be different," she mimics, setting her hand on her hip. "He'll tell me what to buy, what to cook." Her voice falters and I hand her a tissue. "I hate to move. It's a good school system and the teachers are tuned into Lucy's needs. She's had special tutoring." As we talk I visualize a moth caught in the sticky strands, struggling to fly out, its wings useless. She tells me about a therapist Lucy saw last year. "But it's a long drive from where we live now and gas is pricey."

What can I offer her? "I think you're smart not to get more involved with Tom." I say knowing how options are rarely clear-cut. I listen, realize this is taking a long time, but recognize that my time is all I have to give her. Her caring, competence, and insight are evident; I sense her protective judgment about her kids. I tell her that she's a good mother.

She is quiet for a moment and then says, "Not everyone agrees with you."

My heart aches for her. If only I could prescribe a pill that fixes her problems, or cut them out like a diseased organ or a cyst and neatly suture the healthy tissue back together. Because they live in a rural county, fewer services are available to them than if they lived in the city. Luckily they are eligible for Medicaid, which will pay the medical bills and for some counseling. I write down the name of the local food shelf, the hospital social worker and other resources she has not thought of. "You are doing a good job, doing the best you can for the kids," I say and hand her the paper with names and phone numbers.

Lucy and her mother live far enough from my clinic so that I will probably never see them again. Despite this, I will carry them both with me. Carry them and continue to care. Tonight, I will think about them while I plant green onions. And tomorrow, during my morning run, I will mull over their visit, pound into the pavement what I could not do. I cannot remove this boyfriend from their lives. I cannot weave the safety net: find them low incoming housing, create a good job for Lucy's mother, identify competent childcare, locate a good teacher for Lucy, and more. Medical school did not train me to solve the problems of poverty, violence, rural and urban disparities.

Despite the pain of bearing witness, observing the moth struggling in the spider's web, sitting by the wounded, there are gifts that come with my work. I see courage and despair in equal measures. Lucy's mother struggles to care for her kids. Her own needs for intimacy are in conflict with her desire to create a safe home for herself and her children. I watch soberly and wonder if I would be capable of mustering the same courage

I had the guts to leave a bad marriage despite the backlash of some family members who named me scapegoat, but there were no children, only a dog who preceded the marriage. Had there been children, he would have been a good father, a bad husband, but a devoted father, the balance changes. We yearn for simple answers, to paint black and white what is often gray.

Yes, the memory of Lucy and her mother will haunt me. I will pray for them, circle them with white light, and hope that Lucy can plant a different garden, one with more opportunities and less struggle than the one her mother tends. I will dream about this green-eyed girl, wonder how her life unfurls.

Meeting her reminds me to examine what I don't want to see in my own life; I draw lessons from what I witness: suffering, despair, compassion, redemption. We are all struggling. I may have more advantages and resources, but sometimes I am the moth caught in the spider's web. As a fellow human being, there is a measure of guilt in doctoring; I receive more from my patients in humanity than I am ever able to give them.

Lies, White Lies and the Truth

Slats of golden light fell on Sally's hands as she held out her plump and short, pink fingers. A simple gold band encircled her fourth finger. "You know how much I need the pills," she pouted. She was twenty-something with lots of kids, she had endless household chores.

I sat across from her on my stool, mentally preparing myself for her reaction to the accusatory news I needed to deliver. Turning the computer screen toward her, I began. "Your urine drug screen shows no evidence of narcotics. In fact, it shows that you are taking Valium, a medication I'm not giving you. That's a violation of your narcotic contract."

Tears welled, tumbled down her cheeks as she shook her head.

I liked Sally; she'd been my patient for almost three years. She had a rough life: six young children, poverty, depression and pain, but she had a tenacity and resourcefulness I admired. Her husband worked out of town, so much of the time she was a single mom. She had scraped together the money to join the Y. In the evenings she took yoga classes while her kids participated in other activities. Her son with behavior problems loved his dance class; his behavior had improved. Early on, child protection had been involved, but eventually they closed her case. When her children accompanied her to clinic, she seemed to be an attentive mother. She had rheumatoid arthritis and asked me to continue her prescription of Oxycontin. I did.

I am a seasoned physician. When a patient wants narcotics, I request and review old records and make sure that non-narcotic pain medications have been tried. I have patients sign a contract, which outlines the medications and the amounts I agree to give them and the pharmacy where they will fill the prescriptions. I grow suspicious if the patient loses prescriptions, forgets appointments, or asks for additional pills before the designated refill date.

I skimmed Sally's visits to her previous physician. Our narcotic contract limited her to sixty 40 mg tablets of Oxycontin a month, one in the morning and one in the evening. I scheduled an appointment for her with a rheumatologist a few months out. I did not grow suspicious when Sally asked for the smaller 20 mg tablets; she got better results if she staggered them throughout the day. I did not question her when she told me the rheumatologist suggested increasing her dose to five 20 mg tablets daily, although, despite requests, I never received documentation from the rheumatologist. I celebrated with her when child protection rewarded her family with a trip to Disney World.

She always called to cancel an appointment if she could not make it. I only interrogated her briefly when she told me her problem son had dumped all the medications in the medicine cupboard down the toilet. After all, he was a difficult child. I gave her extra Oxycontin for the month. She had only made a request like this once before over the holidays when she had left her medications at her sister's who lived out of state. I was honored when she brought her brother-in-law to see me. But I declined to prescribe Oxycontin for his back pain; his reasons for needing narcotics were unclear and there were no old records documenting his problem.

Two years into my relationship with Sally, the clinic received a fax with details about the Oxycontin prescribed to her address for the past few months. Not only had she paid cash for the last month of Oxycontin, but two other adults in her household were receiving Oxycontin from other physicians. One was the brother-in-law for whom I had refused to prescribe narcotics. She had laid out over $800! How did someone on medical assistance pay $800 cash?

I started doing random urine screens to confirm that Sally was indeed taking her meds. The first screen was positive for Oxycontin, but the second came back negative. After that I confronted Sally, but her excuse seemed believable — she'd run out when she was visiting her Dad in Texas. I gave her the benefit of the doubt. But two months later her second urine drug screen was negative. I could not ignore those results.

"Sally, I can't give you the Oxycontin anymore." I stared at her, setting my jaw.

"But I hurt," Sally blubbered; elephant tears continued to slide down her face.

"Drug tests don't lie," I stated. "You are *not* taking the Oxycontin." I pushed the box of tissue toward her and swallowed my anger. "Let's talk about your depression. Depression hurts too. I can't give you the narcotics, but I can still take care of you." I made an appointment two months out with the new rheumatologist who had started seeing patients at my clinic. "We will see what he says." In the meantime, I rearranged her depression medications and told her to use her Celebrex (a non-narcotic pain medicine) which I had also prescribed for her. She left the clinic crying but returned to her scheduled appointment a month later and asked if I'd reconsider. I declined. We talked about her hectic life and her pain.

I had grown fond of Sally and I'd always enjoyed seeing her. I had been proud of her tenacity and had boasted about her success — my patient with chronic pain who had learned the value of yoga and meditation. I pictured her in the family van filled with kids driving to the Y in the evenings after dinner. Or at least that was what she had told me. Was that a lie as well?

Now, embarrassed that she had bamboozled me, I felt stupid. How much of what she had told me were lies? Twenty years in practice and I'd missed the clues. For three years.

I flagellated myself with *shoulds*:

> I should have reviewed the old visits to her previous physicians more carefully. I did after the fact and clearly saw the clues I'd missed.

> I should have insisted on receiving a copy of the report from the rheumatologist who recommended increasing her dose.

> I should have done urine screens from the beginning.

Sally served as a reminder for me to slow down, be more thorough, spend the additional time with patient records in the evenings after clinic to make sure that all was in order. Always check random urines on patients taking narcotics. My Catholic upbringing had schooled me in *shoulds* and sin.

***

The chalk squealed on the blackboard as Sister Saint Joseph wrote *right and wrong*. The folds of her black veil and floor-length habit swished as she turned to face the class. She brushed white chalk dust from her palms. Only her eyes, mouth and hands seemed alive; the rest of her body was hidden in the pleats and folds of her black habit. "You will be making your first Confession. You are old enough to know the difference." Then beneath *wrong* she printed *sin: mortal, venial.* "Who can tell me the difference?"

My bony arm, stretched up and out of the short-sleeve of my white Peter Pan collared uniform blouse. I'd done my homework at the family dinner table the evening before. My mother, father and I had reviewed my homework questions, as my five younger siblings listened with interest. I was ready.

Sr. Saint Joseph stepped toward the class and scanned the forty squirming second graders. A large rosary swung from the thick black belt at her waist. The beads clinked as she called, "Therese?"

"Venial is little, like telling a lie or pinching my sister. And mortal is big, like killing someone," I said, with confidence, but not too much confidence. Pride was not a good thing. Pride was one of the seven deadly sins.

"Very good, Therese. Thank you. Now class, close your eyes and think about what sins you have committed."

I covered my eyes and tallied them up: I'd argued with and pinched my sister. What else? Someone behind me farted; several students giggled. Through my fingers I saw Sr. Saint Joseph frown in their direction.

We learned that there was right and wrong, big wrongs and little wrongs. Behaviors and thoughts were either good or bad. Sin was doing or thinking bad things. It separated us from God. If we confessed our sins, we could be forgiven and reconnected with God's grace. It was as simple as that. We should always try to do what Jesus would do. Sr. Saint Joseph did not lecture us on the subtle gradations of gray.

I was seven years old, designated the "age of reason," when I made the sacrament of First Confession. I entered the confessional, a closet-sized space off the side aisle of the church and knelt down on the hard kneeler. Amidst darkness and the smell of oiled wood, the priest slid back a little door. Although the screen separated us, I could see his shadow.

"Tell me your sins, my dear." He had stale breath.

I swallowed hard, squeezed my folded hands. I recalled my list. "Fighting with my sister. Sassed back to my mother . . . " There were others, but did I need to confess them? Were they sins? Already I'd begun to wrestle with the gradations of gray.

"Anything else?" the priest queried.

"No Father."

"Say ten *Hail Marys* and listen to your parents." Then he rattled off a prayer too fast for me to understand and finished with, "I absolve you . . ."

I touched my fingers to my forehead and down, around to my shoulders, the sign of the cross. The wooden door squeaked and the priest's shadow disappeared. I found the doorknob, scrambled out of the confessional and into a nearby pew. I pressed my hands together, bowed my head and recited the prayers of my penance. *Hail Mary full of grace . . . Holy Mary Mother of God pray for us sinners.*

***

Sins? What about the gradations between black and white? Were the white lies, some version of the truth or misrepresentation to spare another's feelings?

I can't come to play with Veronica because I have a sore throat. Of course, I didn't have a sore throat. I didn't like Veronica. She smelled and her house was messy, but I couldn't tell her that. A sin? A lie, but a little lie, a shade of the truth.

***

In my own dealings with people I have come to prefer the truth. Just tell me what you are thinking. No sugar-coating. Don't protect me. Don't spare my feelings. Lay your cards on the table. But even now, I am not sure I could say to Veronica: I don't want to come over because you and your house smell.

At work, I know that patients tell me shades of the truth, dole out portions of events and occurrences. Perhaps it is what they think I want to hear, or the reality is too complicated to explain.

Joe told me he was taking his blood pressure medicine. But I was growing convinced that he was not. He was on too many meds, and his blood pressure should have been under better control. Instead of believing him and increasing his dose, I poked around for the truth. "Joe, is it a money problem?" At least he had insurance, but maybe the co-pays were too high? Or "are you having trouble remembering?" He was disorganized; there were competing demands, perhaps a lower blood pressure just wasn't a priority? He could not feel the impact of his high blood pressure? Maybe there were side effects and Joe was too embarrassed to tell me? "Joe, are you worried about your erection?" He stared at his scuffed brown work boots. Maybe that was it. If I knew the whole truth, we could figure out how to proceed. I am not a mind reader, but I am skilled at asking the right questions to get at the truth.

Patients drop clues like bread crumbs. If am paying attention, they lead me to the unvarnished truth. But with Sally I hadn't been paying full attention and my affection for her had clouded my judgment.

***

After the confrontation, Sally checked in with me periodically, but missed many of her scheduled appointments. She kept her appointment with the rheumatologist who diagnosed her with fibromyalgia and declined her request for narcotics. She was angry with him, "He did not spend much time with me." Reports from her insurance company indicated that she'd visited other physicians in the area requesting Oxycontin. Since I was her designated primary care physician, I denied payment for those claims. I talked with child protection about reopening her case. They considered and declined; I did not have evidence that she was a bad mother.

I talked with the clinic lawyer to see if I could report to the police my suspicions about her selling, but due to HIPAA (Health Insurance Portability and Accountability Act) I could not.

Four months later an article in the local paper confirmed my suspicions: Sally and her husband were charged with drug prescription fraud. I had no doubt that Sally was guilty; I'd eventually seen the evidence, even though I'd missed the early clues, partly too busy, partly biased by my affection for Sally. I had trusted her.

***

With my patients I am both the confessor and the accuser. Sometimes I hear the whole truth, every detail as if they must unburden themselves, confess the transgressions, the infidelities, the excesses, the poor judgments that hurt them as well as their loved ones. There is a relief that follows laying bare one's soul. *Here I am and here it is—the awful truth.* As the listener, I must try to accept it without judgment. Personally, I've known that relief, like the clear air after a dramatic summer thunderstorm -- I am washed clean; I can breathe easier; the humidity has vanished.

But I can set patients up to lie. "Joe, you are taking your meds, aren't you?" How could he say no?

It is better to poke around the white lies, to discover the unspoken truth, to ask in a nonjudgmental manner to get at the truth. Sometimes it is embarrassing to admit the facts — I could not bring myself to tell Veronica she smelled as a child. Could I, as an adult, a doctor? *Veronica, I like you. Here is a gift of soap. You'll smell better if you use it. Maybe your mother did not teach you about bathing regularly?* As her physician I could do that, but could I as her friend?

And then, with patients like Sally I missed the clues, perhaps lied to myself for a myriad of reasons. After the fax from the pharmacy the truth could not be avoided: $800 in cash paid when she had insurance? All the other excuses were now so clear in hindsight: Social services paid for Disney World? Did her son really flush her pills down the toilet? How could she run out of her medications and not go through withdrawal?

I became the accuser. I had no choice but to be the accuser.

To be honest, I prefer the role of confessor. It suits my personality more. But as a physician I must be capable of both.

Shining Light in Dark Places

Officer Jerry hands me the digital camera. "Please take pictures of his bottom. He was paddled with a skillet."

I grimace and examine the camera. "Pretty straight forward," I say. Officer Jerry nods; he'd called me earlier that morning to tell me there was a child abuse case that needed documentation. I asked him to come just before lunch so we'd have enough time. I never wanted to rush a child through this type of examination.

I glance at the chart, a seven-year-old boy; the last name is familiar. The fact that I know the family causes me to pause. I've cared for Nicholas's step-mom, collected Pap smears, treated anxiety, and prescribed birth control. I've asked her about domestic violence, several times, which she always denies. I've never met Nicholas, but his father has brought some of the younger children in for immunizations. In this small rural community, I've seen Dad pushing the youngest in the stroller down Main Street. The preschooler pedaled a tricycle alongside and the kindergartner rode a two-wheeler with training wheels. Now this.

The nurse puts Nicholas in the minor procedure room so we wouldn't be crowded and I'd have a good light. The social worker sits on a chair next to a sandy-haired boy who sits tailor fashion on the gurney, his bottom perched on a pillow. He colors a page in a Mickey Mouse coloring book, which is spread out on the surgical tray in front of him.

"Hello Nicolas," I say. "I'm Dr. Zink. I hear that you have some owies that I need to check."

Nicolas looks up and gives me a shy smile. He rolls a thick purple crayon across the tray.

"Tell me what happened last night," I say, pulling up a stool in front of him.

"It's okay," the social worker says putting a hand on his shoulder. "She's here to help you."

Nicolas puts down his crayon and stares at me with a matter of fact expression. "I was bad. My dad spanked me."

"Tell me about the spanking," I say and mentally slip on my yellow rain coat; the compassion can get through, but I won't absorb the negativity.

"On my bottom. It hurts." Nicolas tells me that his Dad paddled him with a skillet. I don't ask what he did. It really doesn't matter. I focus on Nicolas and search for the words to ask the questions I need to ask in a way that will not frighten him or make him a victim again.

"My mouth is sore too."

"Tell me about that."

"I said something bad when I got home from school. Dad put the soap in my mouth then."

How long did you have the soap in your mouth?" I ask. I could see small tears at the corners of his lips.

"I was allowed to take it out for dinner," he says. "We had pizza. It burned."

He fingers the crayons on his tray. His face wrinkles as in the comics when someone is thinking. "Then I had to put it in again until I went to bed."

"What time was that?" I ask.

"About 7:30."

I hear the nurse sigh behind me. I do the math. Home from school about three, out for pizza, maybe an hour if we're lucky, then back in until bedtime, three or four hours.

"How did you sleep last night?" I ask steadying my voice.

Nicolas shrugs his shoulders and I learn that he slept in the stairwell between the first floor and basement as part of his punishment. The social worker's eyes grow wide as Nicolas describes camping under the stairs with his pillow and blanket. Thankfully, the kitchen door to the stairwell and basement was left open. I wonder about his step-mom, if she intervened. And the other children, all younger, where were they?

The horror sits lodged in the back of my throat, I want to cough it up and out. Horror at what people do to people they love. And yet, though I don't have kids, I've met the child abuser in myself, caring for a niece who would not stop whining for her parents. Nothing I did would reassure her and the whine grated like nails on a chalkboard. I know every parent, every adult for that matter, has the capacity to hurt the child who won't stop nagging, crying, just won't stop.

The social worker explains that Nicholas has been living with his dad and step-mom and their three children for the last few months. Before he stayed with his mom in a nearby town and attended a different school. Now I understand why I've not met Nicholas before, but it isn't clear why he moved away from his mother to live with his father and step-mother.

I take a deep breath and begin the most delicate part of the interview: "Did anyone touch you in your private parts," I ask pointing to my own genital area.

Nicolas shakes his head, his blonde bangs flap on his forehead and he stares at his lap.

The social worker leans forward, places a hand on Nicolas's shoe and adds, "It's important to tell the doctor, even if someone told you not to tell. The doctor can help you."

"No one hurt me there," Nicolas says keeping his gaze down.

"Good. I would want to know if they did," I say. I ask the social worker if she has any other questions. She asks if he's been punished like this before and Nicolas affirms that he's been spanked in the past.

I explain to Nicolas that I need to check to see where he is hurt. I tell him that we need to take some pictures of his owies because his dad should not have paddled him so hard. I ask him to move to the side of the cart and he winces as he scoots forward. First, I examine his mouth. His cheeks and tongue are red and the top layer of skin is abraded off inside his mouth next to the corners of his lips. "Does your mouth hurt?" I ask, feeling the lump in my throat again.

"Sort of." He tells me he was able to eat lunch, but the juice burned.

I take photos of his mouth asking him to lift his upper and lower lips for me. He giggles at me as I demonstrate on myself. Handing the camera to the nurse, I methodically look at his ears and neck. There is comfort in the routine, searching for bruises or burns, I examine his arms and torso and visualize every inch of skin; lifting the gown from the sections I need to see and then covering them. The yellow-green bruises I find on his shins are older and starting to heal, probably from play. His feet dangle; his scuffed gym shoes chop the air.

The purple starts at the base of his spine. I position him on his side and have him curl up in a fetal position, bending his knees and draping the sheet to cover him. I swallow a scream as I lift the sheet and take in the bruise that is Nicolas's bottom, a watercolor of blue and purple paint. Anger! It boils through my blood and the camera

24

feels slippery in my sweaty palms. Anger, no, rage, at how Nicholas's father has punished him. Spanking is controversial, but this is over the top.

I frame Nicholas's bottom in the viewer on the back of the digital camera and push the button. Flash, the camera illuminates the bruise. Was his father disciplined like this as a child? Does he only do what he knows? Will his father get the help he needs to learn how to parent differently? Will there be a positive or negative outcome from my efforts? The camera recalibrates and I change the angle slightly and push the button again. I document the injuries, the dark side of human life, what one person can do to another, what an adult has done to a child.

At least one out of ten U.S. children is a victim of abuse, physical and sexual, or neglect, when basic needs such as housing, food, clothing, education, and access to medical care are not provided. Abuse is more common in stressed families, more common with poverty; but no socio-economic stratum is immune. As a physician, I am mandated to report the abuse and neglect of children and seniors. My job is to document what I see and hear, then it is in the hands of the courts. Often, I don't know the outcomes. Sometimes, due to overburdened social services, my reports fall on deaf ears. Will these efforts make a difference today?

Two more photos and then we are done, I tell myself. Flash. Flash.

"Nicolas, you can get dressed," I say, relieved to be done. I high five him, thank him for his help and promise him stickers.

In the hall I flip through the photos with Officer Jerry, again horrified at what I've just witnessed, but I maintain my professional demeanor. "These are great," he says and thanks me.

Great, great photos of *abuse*, but I know what he means. We agree that he will pick up the paper work at 3 p.m. The social worker will take Nicholas to a foster home and I suggest that she instruct them to bring him back if they have any concerns.

The adrenaline has petered out and I push myself to complete the documentation in Nicholas's chart before I take my lunch break. Methodically I type the note into the computer, print it out, and draw the bruises on a body map — a front and back, black and white outline of a child's face and body on an 8 x 11 piece of white paper. All the papers are sealed in a manila envelope for Officer Jerry.

Usually I go for a run over the noon hour and today I am especially eager to do so. The back door of the clinic slams behind me and my shoes slap the asphalt. I pound out the previous hour, sledge hammer to stake. Following a bike trail, I run past fields with corn and soybeans. Harvest has begun in some fields; colossal tractors blow up clouds of dust. Other fields are silent, expectant, the crops bake in the late autumn sun. Breath after breath I huff out the black and blue images. Sweat dampens my armpits and spine, leaking out the poison.

My morning with Nicholas ripples through the afternoon as I wearily minister to another dozen patients, each with an ache, fever or worry. The memory of his blue and purple bottom haunts me and I silently mutter prayers for Nicholas. As the last patient leaves the exam room, I hang my white coat and stethoscope on the hook behind my office door and head home. The rest of my chart notes can wait until morning.

At home I yank off my clothes and step into the steamy shower. Heat. Soap. I rub the bar of soap on my arms, chest, and stomach. I scrub my skin with my loofa and reach behind my shoulder blades and back scouring with a washcloth. When every inch of skin is clean, I wet my hair and lather until I have created an afro of suds. Bending forward at the waist I perform a yoga cleansing breath, pulling air into my abdomen and rolling those muscles up and down, up and down, I exhale with force. I repeat this five times. Dizzy, I anchor myself on the shower stall tile and rinse off, running my fingers through my hair and across by body. Skin stinging, I towel off as I watch the bubbles circle the drain and whisper a prayer for Nicholas and his family. We all have the capacity to be abusers and hazard being victims; may they receive what they need to heal.

I pull on my flannel nightgown and cinch the belt of my robe around my waist. Before making dinner I plug in the tiny white Christmas lights that drape the windows in my living room. I leave them up all year to brighten the late fall and winter nights and tonight I am thankful for their tiny luminescence.

***

Several weeks later, Nicholas's foster-mother brings one of her other children into the clinic. I inquire about how Nicholas has adjusted to his new home. She tells me that initially, he had some trouble getting to sleep at night, but now he's adjusted and seems to enjoy the company of her other children. "He helps one of the younger ones color in our color books," she says. I smile, remembering how fervently he colored here and wonder what shadow the abuse will cast in his life.

Shortly after, that the nurse who assisted me with Nicholas hands me a newspaper and points to the article describing the conviction of Nicholas's father. He will spend several months in jail. A few weeks later I see Nicholas's step-mother and ask her how she is doing at home alone with her three children, now a single parent. "How is your anxiety?"

"I'm getting used to being on my own," she says. "There are advantages, you know." She tells me that she continues to see her therapist.

Again I ask her if her husband, Nicholas's father, ever hurt her.

"I wouldn't let him hit me," she says. "I'm bigger."

I decide not to ask her what she had done during Nicholas's punishment. But she agrees to sign a release so I can talk with her therapist. The therapist tells me that step-mom was present during Nicholas's abuse. "During the episode she froze," the therapist tells me. "She relived what she witnessed as a child and was incapacitated."

***

Even today as I write this, a slight nausea rises in my stomach. After twenty years in practice, I have not acclimated to witnessing this dark side of life. Fortunately, it presents infrequently, but the horror is the same, as sharp and piercing as an ice pick. If I can only shine some light into the darkness, do my part to halt the intergenerational nature of abuse. I inquire, make the report and hope it will make a difference. I am less attached to the outcome, more tolerant of the overburdened social service system. Progress seems to be measured in teaspoons.

***

Nicholas's father is now out of jail. I saw him pushing the stroller down Main Street with his kids the other day. It was a sunny spring day. T-shirt weather. Spring slips into summer quickly in Minnesota. The toddler was in the stroller, another walked alongside holding on to the stroller's rail. The third child pedaled behind. I drove by, then looked in the other direction.

Antibiotics, Por Favor

The afternoon sun streams through the windows of the exam room in the newly refurbished Rochester Migrant Clinic. The walls show no hint of wear or tear and the exam table still holds remnants of plastic wrap. I have explained to the señora and her daughter why it is not good to treat viral infections with antibiotics. They jabber in Spanish, hands flying. The señora's gray hair is pulled into a taut bun, emphasizing the lines of living in her face. Her calloused hands speak of pounding corn, flattening tortillas, and cleaning. A bleached-white apron corsets her bosom and abdomen and hides her floral patterned dress. The daughter, a younger version of her mother, wears a stylish blouse and slacks. Her gray roots are concealed by orange-brown hair-dye.

The interpreter translated my several-minute explanation into one sentence — something got lost. The women's expressions are somber and their voices hiss with dissatisfaction. Now they are questioning the interpreter. I understand words and phrases. The conversation stops and the interpreter says to me: "She wants a penicillin injection."

My heart sinks. Helping patients understand why the common cold should not be treated with antibiotics is exhausting. Often it would be easier just to give them what they want. After years of receiving antibiotics for most maladies, patients are disappointed when I won't prescribe them. The rapidly increasing number of organisms that are antibiotic resistant has spawned an international effort to limit the use of antibiotics. However, patients still expect them, especially patients from other countries, such as Latin America where antibiotics can be purchased over the counter.

Even non-immigrant U.S. born patients expect antibiotics. Older patients in my regular clinic have told me: "In the old days Doc Smith just gave me a penicillin shot for my cold. I got better quick." And the long-time patients of my colleague assume that I'll prescribe antibiotics like he does. Some snort their disgust when I say no and I steel myself as they reply, "I'll just call Dr. Allen tomorrow." Perhaps my patient satisfaction scores would be higher if I complied, but then I'd be contributing to the already burgeoning antibiotic resistance. I've drawn my line.

The señora reports having a stuffy nose, cough, and sore throat for two days, but no fever. Antibiotics are not indicated -- and definitely not a penicillin injection. With a deep breath, I shove my frustration aside and try again. I ask the interpreter to translate each sentence:

"Penicillin doesn't treat viral infections."

"If I give you a penicillin shot, it will make your hip sore and help the bacteria grow stronger."

"Your body can fight the virus on its own."

"Get rest. Drink lots of liquids."

I talk about using acetaminophen or ibuprofen and returning for a recheck next week if she is not better.

The señora's frown deepens, her daughter shakes her head.

"Lo siento mucho, señora. Regrese usted en una semana," I say recalling my month of Spanish immersion in Mexico three months earlier. My Spanish improved, but not as much as I'd hoped. I still could not have a complex conversation with a patient on my own. I'd lived with a family and we spoke only Spanish. Mornings I observed at the Cruz Rojo (Red Cross) clinic for the poor and

uninsured. Afternoons were spent doing Spanish grammar drills with my *maestra* (teacher).

As I walked through the swinging doors into the Cruz Rojo clinic, the familiar smell of ammonia greeted me, the pungency strikes me the same, causing my eyes to water, no matter where I've doctored. Despite its cleanliness, the facility exhibited the slightly beleaguered appearance of many Latin American medical centers -- scuffed walls, frayed gurneys with no paper on them, and medical supplies locked in a central location. Nurses wore white pants suits and nursing students dressed in starched red-and-white striped uniforms with white caps perched on their heads. Staff greeted each other by brushing cheek against cheek or lips. My personal space alarm bells shrieked when the administrator of Cruz Rojo acknowledged me this way after having met me only once. Eventually, I learned to do as the Mexicans.

Dr. Roberto, the Urgent Care physician at Cruz Rojo, was dark-skinned with acne scars on his face and a protruding belly. He spoke little English, but he was patient with my efforts to speak Spanish and gently corrected my pronunciation. In return, he asked me to enunciate a medical diagnosis in English, then he'd practice it the rest of the morning: seizure, seizure, emphasis on the *zure*. Like many U.S. physicians, he draped his stethoscope around his neck and wore a white coat with his name embroidered in red on the pocket. A physician at the clinic for ten years, his seniority allowed him to work only the day shift. His younger colleagues, who rotated shifts, flirted with the nurses and had little time for me. Since Dr. Roberto was genuinely interested in helping me, I shadowed him. He introduced me to patients as: *"Doctora Teresa vive en Estados Unidos. Estudia Español para ayudar los inmigrantes de México."*

Pharmaceutical representatives from the same companies that had called on me in the U.S. visited Dr. Roberto and left samples, shiny pamphlets, journal reprints, pens, and pads of paper with logos. Nurses and doctors shared treats—*dulces and papas fritas*-- carried in their pockets from the break room or hidden in drawers at the nurse's station. As in the U.S., nurses set up and cleaned up after the doctors. Carefully arranged on the tray were the pack of sterile gloves, the lidocaine already drawn up in the syringe, and a pile of gauze sponges. When done with a procedure, the doctors ripped off their gloves and ignored the disarray they had created.

When a patient was ready for evaluation, a half sheet of computer-generated paper appeared in the box hanging on the door of the intake office. Dr. Roberto picked up the paper, walked to the waiting area and called the patient into his office. The patient was typically accompanied by a family member, and they were invited to sit in the hard-back chairs across from Dr. Roberto's desk. A computer, opened to a web-based pharmaceutical desk reference, sat on his right. Across the room, an exam table that wore the same paper sheet for days paralleled the wall. Pharmaceutical samples were kept in the unlocked closet. The bathroom where he fastidiously washed his hands between patients opened next to the closet.

I sat or stood next to the patient. Dr. Roberto invited the patient to describe symptoms, then asked questions. If I could organize my Spanish words into what I wanted to say, I also posed questions. Then Dr. Roberto performed an exam and handed me his stethoscope or flashlight so that I could do the same. He religiously checked throats and rarely looked in ears. If there were abdominal complaints, he palpated the abdomen. Often he asked me what I thought: *"Tratamiento?"*

I tiptoed around the differences in our approaches. In the U.S. we always looked in the ears of children and were less concerned about throats in toddlers younger than two years. Despite patients' requests for antibiotics for a cold or viral infection, I refrained from prescribing them despite their disappointment. In contrast, Dr. Roberto treated them with an antibiotic and at least three other pills (one for cough, another for congestion, acetaminophen or Ibuprofen for discomfort). Abdominal complaints were also treated with antibiotics and an antispasmodic medicine, usually given through an intravenous line.

Dr. Roberto carefully wrote prescriptions and instructions on a single half sheet of paper with the Cruz Rojo emblem, stamped his title and then scrawled his signature. The directions included symptomatic treatments such as drink liquids, avoid caffeine or *refrescos* (soda pop), and rest. Prescriptions were purchased at the Cruz Rojo pharmacy that was more economical than the other private pharmacies. He encouraged patients to return in a few days for a recheck. "Patients love their Penicillin injections and antibiotics," Dr. Roberto told me. "In Mexico they can buy them from any pharmacy without a prescription."

When we discussed the treatment of a patient, I highlighted the similarities and cautiously explained our differences. The antibiotic issue was a challenge. As an example, I described the rapid strep test to Dr. Roberto. Studies had shown that physicians were not particularly good at distinguishing strep from other viral throat infections. By swabbing the throat, then placing the swab in reagents for five to ten minutes, the rapid strep test provided a highly sensitive indication of whether or not the patient had strep growing in his or her throat. The test had greatly reduced the use of antibiotics for pharyngitis in the U.S.

Dr. Roberto was impressed and asked, "*Cuanta cuesta?*"

"About $25 per test-kit," I said.

"*Muy caro!*" he exclaimed. And by Mexican standards this was expensive.

One afternoon, I went to a pharmacy to practice my Spanish and to check the availability of certain drugs. Twelve 500 mg tablets of Amoxicillin cost approximately $6 U.S. At home, I usually prescribed twenty for strep throat, costing just under $12, or half of the price of the rapid strep test.

To put this in perspective, a Mexican who worked at McDonald's in Mexico and was employed part-time, received no health benefits and made $1 U.S. an hour. He or she would need to work 25 hours to pay for the rapid strep test and half that to pay for the Amoxicillin.

Despite his willingness to give patients what they wanted, Dr. Roberto was worried about antibiotic resistance. He had heard the messages of the international campaigns: treatable illnesses become untreatable. We talked about *las problemas con resistencia a antibióticas* and *fuerte bacteria*. Why did he continue to give antibiotics for what was clearly a viral infection? In the U.S. some doctors continued to prescribe antibiotics in the face of other recommendations; changing behavior was hard. Was Dr. Roberto pleasing patients or was I missing something?

During my residency (family medicine specialty training), I cared for Hmong patients, immigrants from Laos who had settled in St. Paul, Minnesota, after the Vietnam War. I'd never encountered this population before. One day, I examined a child and noticed a line of bruises on his back, circular reddish or purple hued spots about three inches wide. Worried, I asked the attending physician why the parents abused their sick child. "This is cupping or coining," he said and explained the custom. Hot cups or coins were applied to the skin to draw out the fever or bad humors that caused illness.

Was there some cultural issue in Mexico related to antibiotics? I mulled this over for several days and while pouring a glass of purified water from the dispenser at my family's home, an idea occurred to me. Not drinking the water from the faucet was stressed by my housemother and in papers from the school. Folks with money, like my host family, purchased 10-gallon jugs of purified water. But the poor would not have the resources for this. In the clinic, stomach cramps were a common complaint. The next day I asked Dr. Roberto about this and he confirmed the *contaminación del agua*. Dr. Roberto usually prescribed a Ciprofloxacin equivalent and an injection for spasms of the colon. Perhaps he was treating a bacterial problem. However, in the U.S. we refrained from using antibiotics for diarrhea unless there was blood in the stool, a fever, or copious diarrhea.

I realized that something about our differences did reach Dr. Roberto when he asked me to explain our practices in the U.S. at the monthly staff meeting. Physicians and nurses gathered around a large table in the center of the conference room where paintings of local city scenes hung on the walls. A breeze blew through the open windows. After presenting the case of an adolescent who had died from a severe reaction to a scorpion bite, Dr. Roberto opened the floor to other topics of concern. The head nurse brought up the issue of giving injections to patients without prescriptions. Because patients could purchase injections and syringes over the counter, they sometimes came to the urgent care asking a nurse to administer the shot. Dr. Roberto railed on for five minutes about not providing this service, then he turned to me and asked me to explain the necessity of prescriptions for many medications in the United States.

In my hesitant Spanish, I talked about the fact that most medications like antibiotics, anti-hypertensives, birth control pills and medicines for diabetes required a prescription and how even the syringes for insulin couldn't be purchased without a prescription. As a result, in the United States patients could only receive an injection through the order of a physician. Dr. Roberto repeated what I had said, translating my Spanish into Spanish. I smiled to myself; at least I understood everything he said.

***

Now at the Rochester Migrant Clinic, I face the Mexican señora and her daughter. Their scowls carve deep furrows in their brows. Their years of medical care in Mexico have taught them that good care means pills, several types of pills and sometimes injections. For this illness, they have received only words of reassurance. Graciously, they take my hand and thank me, but I hear them commiserate in Spanish, shaking their heads as they walk out the door. The interpreter, a younger woman, smiles at me and shrugs her shoulders. We watch them leave with their confidence in the medicine they have always known as strong as ever. I stand alone with my impotence. So much was needed; so little I could do.

Second Guessing the Second Opinion

"Dobre dien, sleepy head." Jeffrey woke me from a Sunday afternoon nap. An American and the director of our project, Jeffrey was a fluent Russian speaker. "Nazir and his wife are upstairs with their son. They want you to examine him."

Where was I? It came back quickly -- on an international aid mission with Doctors Without Borders in Chechnya. We supplied Chechen physicians in war-torn hospitals with medications and equipment. Physicians shared data about the illnesses and injuries they were treating, including the numbers of landmine and gunshot victims. As a result, we had the most complete data about the impact of the Russian-Chechen struggle. We shared this with both international agencies and human rights organizations. Restless with my privileged American life I'd come for an adventure and to do some good. However, I'd begun to wonder if I could make any difference.

I trudged up the outside stairs to the office. The afternoon air was chilly; the sun low in the cloudless sky cast a golden light. The neighbor's dog barked again. From the second floor porch, I could see the steel gray, snow-capped and craggy Caucasus Mountains, the backbone of this region.

Nazir was one of my favorite guards. He often helped me with my pronunciation when I studied my Russian and rode the exercise bike in our makeshift gym, a room that was part storage and the place our Muslim staff came to pray throughout the day. Russian was the common language here, although some staff members spoke Chechen or Ingush with each other. Each evening before supper, Nazir made a quick trip home to administer vitamins to his son. Medical practice was so different here, but staff regularly brought me their "healthy" family members to get the opinion of an "American" doctor. Often I had little to offer because they'd already purchased injectable antibiotics from the pharmacy that would not help their viral infections. Or the inhaler they needed was not available. A different part of the world, but the issues were the same, patients wanted something I could not give -- a pill for something that instead demanded their time and patience or what they really needed was beyond their reach.

I concealed a yawn and greeted Nazir who stood proudly next to his petite wife who held their son, Sasha, my patient. Behind them cabinets built to hold china and crystal were stuffed with binders of data. Three computers sat on three of the six desks.

Eighteen-month-old Sasha struggled to climb out of his mother's arms. Her henna-dyed hair was pulled back from her forehead and covered with a red headscarf that coordinated with her checkered dress. Gold buttons that matched her earrings marched down the front bodice. Sasha fingered them, then wiggled and babbled pointing toward the wall with windows. When she set him down on the wooden floor, he toddled between the metal desks and office chairs to the large windows that opened to the street a story below. Good motor development for his age. His mother followed after him, her high-heeled square-toed boots clicked on the floor boards. Sasha clutched the window ledge with his fat hands and jabbere -- appropriate language for his age.

Nazir explained his child's health problems in Russian and Jeffrey translated. "Their child had problems at birth. I'm not exactly sure what. He was in the hospital for two weeks."

This was not terribly long. In Russia and Eastern Europe, healthy moms and babies remained in the hospital for a week, a stark contrast to the 24-hour hospital stays in the U.S. Jeffrey handed me the child's medical records — a dozen stapled scraps of paper covered with blue and black Cyrillic letters. As I flipped through, my frustration flared, lots of numbers in no particular order, no graphs.

Jeffrey continued, "The doctors monitor him regularly, as these records show. Nazir gives him vitamin injections to aid his growth."

I gasped and interrupted. "Where does he give the injections?"

"In the legs."

Shivers erupted along my spine at the thought of a needle shoved into the thigh muscle of his young boy, and every day. I'd known that Nazir ran home, but seeing his child I remembered the slides of crippled children during a medical lecture a year or so ago. In Eastern Europe, children had become lame because of frequent injections in the legs. Some component of the preservative probably atrophied the muscles. I watched Sasha waddle around the room; he was lucky, so far.

"Now the doctors want to give him some kind of brain medicine." Jeffrey handed me a slip of paper with scribbled Russian.

I took a deep breath and marched over to the cabinet reaching for the Russian *Physician Desk Reference*. The book was the same size as the PDR in the U.S. Our computer access was erratic so checking the internet was not a reliable option. Sounding out the letters I pronounced the name -- foreign to me. I'd learned the phonetics of the Cyrillic letters and could sometimes recognize words. Because most medical terms had a Latin root, I could usually figure out enough of the meaning to understand the significance. If not, Jeffrey, despite his non-medical background, was always interested in helping.

"Looks like it's for dilation of the blood vessels Is that what you're reading?" I asked.

Jeffrey looked over my shoulder and mumbled, "Vessels in the brain to be specific."

"It's oral?"

Nazir confirmed that this new medicine was to be taken by mouth and that the vitamin injections were to be continued.

Folding my arms I presented the dilemma to Jeffrey. "We had nothing like this for kids in the U.S. This medicine must be expensive. And they pay out of pocket." There was no health insurance. Since the Russian invasion of Chechnya and the Chechens' victory, of sorts, the Soviet infrastructure had crumbled. And the vitamin injections could damage the muscles, not to mention injury to the nerve if Nazir placed the injection in the wrong place. What about the cleanliness of the needles? Needles and syringes might be purchased from vendors on the street; how well were they sterilized? I'd dipped my toe into a morass. There were no easy answers here.

I began with the familiar."Will you ask Mom to hold Sasha while I examine him?" There was a comfort with this routine. First, we laid him on a desk to measure his height, then his head circumference. We didn't have a scale, but he was not malnourished. I charted the results on a growth chart that I'd brought with me and finished the exam: looked in his eyes, ears, and mouth, palpated his neck, listened to his lungs and heart. Sasha laughed when I felt his stomach. His genitals were normal. This was a healthy child.

I handed Jeffrey the blue growth chart, which graphed age appropriate height and weight for boys. "See how I graphed his measurements. I would expect to see something like this." I pointed to the ink dots on the chart. "Instead they've written down numbers almost weekly. Look at these dates. The numbers don't seem to have any progression. I question their accuracy. A lot of hassle and worry for Nazir and his wife -- lots of doctor visits. How do I tell them this physician is a crock?" I searched Jeffrey's face.

They wanted my advice, but Jeffrey had worked in the area for over five years, overseeing various projects in the North Caucasus. I'd been here a couple of months and was still negotiating the cultural disconnect. Physicians had their ways of doing things and were proud and resistant to changes. During the years of the Soviet Union, medical practice was isolated from the burgeoning medical knowledge in the rest of the world.

Jeffrey gave me a mischievous grin. "You're the doctor."

Right now, I wanted help, not humor. I wished he'd give me the right answer. Was there a right answer? What did Nazir and his wife really need from me? In this small town their physician would be their doctor for years to come. Could I say he was a quack? Do they have other options? Frequent injections could be crippling. I'd never heard of this brain medicine and I was not sure that Sasha needed it. Everything cost money. He was a healthy child. His parents needed to feed and nurture him and stop all the medications and injections. But was I certain about my assessment? I couldn't look at his brain, there was no CAT scan. But his exam was completely normal. Was there something I didn't know, something I was missing? Always a possibility. Why was I second guessing myself?

How did I deal with this cultural quagmire, the different approaches to medical care, my own self doubts? The current treatment could cripple this child. If I shared my concerns, I could make a difference in the life of Nazir's son. But I had to scale my own insecurities; did I trust my assessment enough to say Sasha's doctor was wrong? If so, how did I respect their choices so far and suggest another way? I would only be here for a short period in Sasha's life, less than a year. If he became sick and needed a doctor after I'd left, would their doctor retaliate because they chose not to follow his advice? This was an authoritative culture. I shook my head and looked at Jeffrey. "You're not helping me on this one?"

Jeffrey shrugged.

But I had a responsibility to educate. Their resources were limited; they were wasting their money and possibly harming their child. How did I insert doubt and educate, offer another option. I took a deep breath and watched Sasha scamper from chair to desk to chair.

Then Jeffrey came through. "You could suggest they talk with Dr. Musa."

Dr. Musa was a respected Chechen neurosurgeon now treating primary care problems. As the head Chechen physician for our project, he periodically shadowed me when I saw patients, trying to understand our western ways of practice and to learn the management of primary care problems. As a neurosurgeon he knew how to cut and sew, but not the treatment of diarrhea or asthma. Jeffery had hired him because he was well connected throughout Chechnya.

"Good idea." I could talk with him, explain my apprehensions. "Tell me if this is appropriate." I took a breath. "Based on what I know, your child is normal. This brain medicine does not exist in the U.S. I don't think he needs it. I'm also worried about the vitamin injections. Studies in the U.S. show that they can harm the leg muscles and eventually cripple a child. However, I was not trained here and doctors do things differently. You might talk with Dr Musa. He's smart and may know someone who can help you."

Jeffrey smiled and then translated. Nazir held his son and gently kissed his hair. His wife stood near watching his expression. When

42

Jeffrey finished, Nazir gave me a broad smile, explained things to his wife, then they both thanked me and shook my hand. Here men and women didn't shake the hands of local women, but because I was an American and a physician I have some other status.

"*Spaceba*," his wife said and followed Nazir down the stairs to their car in the courtyard. I watched them climb into their car and realized the importance of trusting what I knew. Self-doubt could be a double-edged knife: knowing my limits and asking for help, knowing what I know and being secure in that. Jeffrey handed me a way to negotiate the cultural overlays. Musa would understand and respect my opinion and could guide Nazir and his family to another local physician should they need help after I left.

Nazir's wife held her son on her lap in the front seat of their white Lada, a Russian model. There were no infant seats and neither Nazir nor his wife fastened their seatbelts. Unfortunately here in Chechnya there were graver dangers.

Field Clinics in Honduras

The new clinic in Pinares, Honduras, has Pepto-Bismol pink trim and a turquoise door--colors that are not unusual in a country where markets are filled with multi-hued fruits and vegetables, and the folks tending them dress in orange, red and royal blue. Their white shirts and blouses are brighter than anything I can achieve with bleach in my washer at home. The clinic was built by a non-profit group in the United States that sponsors a non-government organization in Honduras. A local physician staffs the clinic once a week, and a nurse cares for the patients on the other days. At least twice a year, groups from the U.S. come to provide more intensive medical care for a few weeks.

Several years ago, I served as faculty for one of these groups. We ran a daily clinic in Pinares, held clinics in nearby villages, and visited the homes of patients who could not walk to see us. The mountainous terrain limits agricultural pursuits and transportation, making this one of the more impoverished regions of Honduras. Most people travel by foot; a horse is a luxury.

When we first arrived in Pinares, we met with the clinic's community board, a dozen women and men from the surrounding villages. They explained the assets and challenges of their communities and we scheduled our field clinics.

Mid-week, Luis, the mayor of La Esperanza, a village a couple of hours into the mountains, guided my team into the countryside. The group included Bret, a fourth-year medical student who planned on specializing in internal medicine; Chris, a nursing student and basketball player whose stamina almost equaled that of

Luis, our guide; Jose, our lanky translator, a ninth grader at the English school on the Honduran coast who was making his first trip to this region of his country. He had more in common with members of our group than he did with Luis or the other locals. The women included Linda, a pharmacy student, and Mary, a first-year resident in Family Medicine. This was the first trip to Honduras for everyone in the group except Mary and me. Mary had made a similar trek two years earlier, so she knew what she was in for. At fifty years of age, I was the oldest in the group, but was training for a marathon, so I was in good shape.

Wearing hiking boots, sunglasses and hats, our back packs stuffed with a change of clothes, sleeping bags and medical supplies, we were a stark contrast to Luis who travelled light, scaling the mountain in his sandals like a goat. He never broke a sweat and carried no water. Small and thin, like most Honduran men in this region, and somewhere in his forties, he outpaced everyone, following a narrow rocky path up the mountain and scrambling effortlessly down the backside.

The scenery was spectacular. Craggy rocks covered with pines at the higher elevations, where the locals grew coffee, descended to thick green foliage. Creeks cut through the valleys, and birds called from everywhere in the brush. Butterflies fluttered about, and the occasional blooming bush perfumed the air. In another country, someone would pay big bucks to have a private guide in mountains like these.

Less sure-footed, we picked our way, checking our footing so we didn't slip on patches of scree. My back dripped with sweat, soaking my backpack. Although I needed my long sleeve shirt and hat for sun protection, both grew wet enough to wring out.

We came to a gushing stream where we had two options for crossing: Either balance on a branch about four inches in diameter that served as the foot bridge or take off our boots and wade across, keeping our footing on the slippery rocks in the swiftly flowing water. Once on the other side, we guzzled water, sharing a bottle with Luis, and splashed water from the stream on our faces and necks.

As we descended the mountain, the first village with its tile and corrugated metal roofs appeared in the distance. At the outskirts of the town, the landscape leveled out. On the village's main street, we saw elderly folks gathered near the school waiting for us. Many of the women had aprons tied over their colorful dresses, and both the men and women wore ball caps. We were late, but this was Honduran time. Luis entered the classroom announcing our arrival. The teacher led her noisy class of twenty first through sixth graders into the school yard and across the road, directing them to sit on the church steps. Their antics were quickly hushed as they resumed their lessons.

We rearranged the wooden furniture, turning the classroom into our clinic with two "offices." We set up two chairs and a desk in opposite corners of the room, hoping the distance would create some privacy. Chris carried another desk out to the porch for registration and Linda situated one near the door for our pharmacy. Jose and Mary lined up the extra chairs along the wall on the porch where waiting locals quickly occupied them.

Chris and Jose registered the patients on half-sheet forms, filling in name (usually there were four — two first names and a maternal and paternal last name), village and birth date. Bret and Mary, who both spoke some Spanish, each staffed an exam area and I floated between them, checking out each patient. Women mopped their foreheads with the small towels they carried and flapped them as fans. I relented and opened the avocado green shutters, I'd closed for privacy. During their classroom break, giggling students peered in the windows to watch us.

Prescriptions were written on post-it notes, which patients carried over to Linda. She had a small supply of soap, sunscreen, lotions, ibuprofen, acetaminophen, an anti-depressant, and a few antibiotics, which she tucked into sandwich-size baggies and labeled.

Because most of the people engaged in physical labor and ate a diet of rice and beans and local fruit and vegetables, few had hypertension or diabetes. The elderly patients came with complaints of arthritis, rashes, varicose veins, and toothaches.

We treated the teacher's son who complained of stomach bloating for worms. She coaxed him to drink the strawberry-flavored abendazole. The matron who tended the church asked us to examine her daughter. The thin, twenty-year-old woman looked to be twelve or thirteen. Bret discovered a loud heart murmur — *lub, swosh, dub* -- and clubbed fingernails (the thickened flesh under the nails caused the nails to curve downward, mimicking round part of an upside-down spoon). This suggested low oxygen levels in her blood. We promised to arrange a consultation with a cardiologist at the university in the capital, Tegucigalpa. The organization set aside money to transport patients like her for specialty care. The repair of her heart could add years to her life; modern medicine did have its miracles.

At the end of our session, we repositioned the desks and chairs so the class could resume. Linda videotaped the students during a lesson, and afterward the students circled around her, hooting and pointing as they watched themselves on the camera's screen. The teacher blushed when she saw herself on the video.

We repacked our supplies, waved our farewells and followed Luis to the edge of the village, where we ate peanut butter sandwiches, oranges and cookies in the shade of a smooth-barked *Ceiba* tree.

We made several home visits before our last stop, a wooden shack made of weathered boards with gaps between them. Although the spacing allowed the smoke from the cooking fire to escape, it also let in mosquitoes and flies. Children and chickens ran into the house from the yard. I counted six heads; the youngest, about two years old, sat on the dirt floor without a diaper and played with a mangy looking kitten. Stepping over a small pile of chicken poop, we approached the patient, the *abuela* (grandmother) of this house. She lay on a 2-foot-high wooden platform, cushioned with a thin mattress and several blankets. She sat up and greeted us, smoothing her white blouse and print skirt. Shaking hands with each of us, she then pointed to her knees. They were thick with the boney changes you see with arthritis. The mother of the household rattled on in Spanish to Jose. It seemed that the *abuela*'s right knee was more painful than her left.

"She can't walk," Jose interpreted.

"Is there more?" I asked, not believing that Jose had translated everything the mother had said.

"Not really," Jose said. "She was telling me that her knees have bothered her for a long time and that they painted clay from the creek on her knees to help the pain." Bret and Mary examined her. When they were finished, I asked what they wanted to do.

"Acetaminophen?" Mary suggested.

"We could inject her knee with steroids," I replied. "We have the supplies." I asked if either had done one before. Mary had performed several, but Bret had only watched, so we decided to let him do the procedure. Since Bret would begin an internal medicine residency in the summer, this was a good skill for him to learn.

We pulled our supplies out of our backpacks, opened a pair of sterile gloves and spread the glove paper out on the corner of the bed to create our sterile area. We scrubbed off the dried black clay with water from our canisters, then Bret drew up the mixture of steroid and lidocaine. I showed him how to position the patient with her knee slightly bent and feel for the opening between the knee cap and the end of the upper leg bone. Bret painted the knee with betadine, pulled on the sterile gloves, carefully fingered the spot and inserted the needle. I talked Bret through each step; he performed the procedure like an expert.

With the prick of the needle the *abuela* winced, but the medicine flowed in easily. Some of the older children gathered to watch, whispering among themselves. The *abuela* thanked us as we wiped off the betadine, applied a bandage over the injection site and wrapped her knee with an elastic wrap. She sat up to inspect her knee and bowed her head toward us.

I congratulated Bret on his success and shooed away the small furry black puppy, who'd fallen asleep on his pack during the procedure. We left the family with two bars of soap and toothbrushes. We did not leave toothpaste because we worried that hungry children might eat it. Linda labeled a bag of twenty acetaminophen tablets with the *abuela*'s name and the date. The mother of the household untied a plastic bag from a board that ran underneath the roof, tucking the small pill pack inside. This was typical storage for families, a location that was dry and up and away from children and animals.

The town of Estrella was a 20-minute hike down the mountain. We set up our quarters for the evening in the one-room adobe brick school. We had about an hour until sunset. Since we were near the equator, there were exactly twelve hours of darkness and twelve hours of daylight.

Luis raced off to get our dinners. Several of us gathered water bottles, filled them with cold water that we pumped from the well and purified with my ultraviolet wand. Chris and Jose played soccer with some of the local boys on the dirt field in front of the school with a soccer ball that Chris had carried and planned to leave with the children. One small daredevil darted in at the last minute to kick the ball away from Chris, causing him to tumble. The boys laughed heartily, jumping up and down and slapping each other on the back. Red-faced, Chris stood up, and resumed the game until it began to drizzle.

The smell of rain filled the yard. Soon, a late afternoon cloudburst pelted us and we took shelter under the eve along with the children. Chris removed his shirt and grabbed a bar of soap, lathering under his arms and over his hairy chest. The kids giggled, and a few removed their shirts and mimicked him, so he shared his bar of soap. Bret and Jose joined in, and then the women stripped down to sports bras. Within a few minutes, all of us were lined up at the edge of the porch to catch the water running off the roof. The cold water revitalized me, and the soap cut through the acrid and salty sweat generated by the day.

The drone of the rain on the roof resembled a locomotive coming down the mountain. Suddenly, it was over and we could hear the voices and clatter of our neighbors as they prepared their evening meals. We dug towels out of our packs, dried off, taking turns in the school room to pull on dry clothes. Wet capri's, khaki pants with zip off legs, T-shirts hung over the small wooden chairs and tables.

Drenched, Luis arrived with our dinners, and a large watermelon tied to his back. We lined up chairs on the porch and guiltily devoured our beans, rice, chicken and tortillas. The children eyed us hungrily. We split the watermelon with our pocket knives and handed out slices to a sea of hands. The fruit was sugary sweet.

Standing on the porch, Chris spit his seeds out into the yard. A few of the boys and girls followed his lead, giggling as juice dribbled down their chins.

When it grew dark, I shooed the children away. Inside the school, we turned on our flashlights and unrolled our sleeping bags and pads on the concrete floor.

I settled my head on my fleece vest. In the distance, I could hear the sounds of the night, so different from home. A bird called with an owl-like hoot. Insects chirped. Soft breathing and gentle snores began to surround me.

We rose about 6 a.m., ready for Luis when he arrived with a thermos of hot coffee and tortillas and scrambled eggs wrapped in tin foil. Our sleeping bags were rolled up, our packs stashed in the corner and the school room was transformed into a clinic.

On the porch, I breathed in the crisp morning air, clean and fresh after the evening's rain. The school yard was muddy with scattered watermelon seeds and rinds. A large mango tree, the leaves brilliantly green in the morning sunlight, stood in the far corner. The doctor at the clinic in Pinares had spoken about the increase in broken arms and sprains from kids who climbed the mango trees, scooting far out on the branches to reach the luscious fruits. Luckily, mango season was over before we arrived. A stream of patients made their way toward the school.

"Bret, come see our first patient," I called from the porch. Cautiously finding her footing on the path down the mountain was the *abuela* whose knee Bret had injected the day before. Dressed in the same skirt and blouse and with a wide smile on her face, she leaned on her cane, fashioned from a tree branch. Bret watched her progress, a look of surprise on his whiskered face. When she arrived at the porch, she hugged him, her head barely reaching the middle of his chest.

A thoughtful and quiet young man, Bret said nothing, but grinned, looking toward me. My chest was so tight with joy I felt like it might burst, much like the juicy watermelon we'd sliced open the evening before. Bret talked with his patient; she was feeling so much better that she wanted us to inject her other knee.

Moments like this are to be savored and remembered, one that I have carried with me and replayed: Seeing Bret gaze at the *abuela* picking her way down the mountain. Observing his face and her face, both with broad smiles. Watching the *abuela* step up on to the porch and hug Bret, the kindness in his eyes.

At home, where material goods are plentiful, I forget to appreciate what I can do for patients. In rural Honduras, the impact of my actions is immediate and real. At home, a knee injection is a knee injection. But here, a grandmother who could not walk yesterday could tromp down the mountain today.

Mystery

One cannot help but be in awe when he contemplates the mysteries of eternity, of life, of the marvelous structure of reality. It is enough if one tries merely to comprehend a little of this mystery every day. Never lose a holy curiosity.

Albert Einstein (1879 - 1955)

‡ ‡ ‡

Reborn in Honduras

A car horn blared outside the cement block clinic in Santa Lucia, Honduras, just as we finished our dinner of tortillas, beans and rice. A battered and rusty green car dropped off a young couple at the clinic door. I was on call for the evening along with a nurse, resident physician and a medical and a nursing student. We were visiting the clinic for two weeks for an international health course at an Ohio university. The mother stood at the clinic door clutching a bundled infant. She wore the garb of recent childbirth -- a white cloth turban on her head and cotton stuffed in her ears to keep out the "cold." I recognize her husband; only yesterday I'd removed the sutures from his repaired scalp, a machete wound. The mother handed the baby to me and reached for her husband's hand. Opening the bundle I discovered a gray and floppy infant with shallow respirations, medical parlance for a very sick kid. This baby needed a pediatric intensive care unit; for me that hospital rotation was at least a decade earlier. I told the on-call team to summon the rest of our crew for help and struggled to remember my Spanish, stammering, "*Quantos dias tiene su hijo?*"

"*Once.*" Their baby was eleven days old.

Our team included three family physicians, two dentists, two midwives, four family medicine residents, four fourth-year medical students, and three nursing graduate students. The team was big on enthusiasm and used to "big city" medicine. Half of the group was running a clinic in a village two hours away. The remaining crew was a little bored, deciding what card game to play. This rural Honduran clinic was founded several years earlier by a U.S.

physician who took "the bus to the end of the road" and then worked with the local community to build the clinic. Now, two full-time local physicians staffed the clinic, supported in part with semi-annual visits from University teams to replenish supplies and give the regular doctors a break. Prior to this, a public health nurse and an occasional visiting physician, from Cuba, had provided medical care to the community. Patients had told me that the public health clinic was often out of the government-paid-for medications.

The team worked swiftly. The local physicians stayed in the background, allowing our visiting group to run the show.

Through one of our translators, ninth graders from the well-to-do English school along the coast, we learned that the baby had been delivered by a local birth attendant and had not eaten for four days. Dr. Ed managed the infant's airway with a small mask and an old oxygen concentrator that made up for its lack of efficiency with its noise. Was it effective? Hard to tell. The pediatric nurse practitioner student, a former pediatric intensive care nurse, stepped forward. She attempted to start an intravenous (IV) line in the baby's tiny arm and failed. The dentist/oral surgeon succeeded in the baby's foot. Supplies were found, or creatively adjusted to be appropriate for a baby. Glucose was added to a saline IV bag. Antibiotics were given through the IV.

Someone located the dusty leather suitcase that contained medications for resuscitations. Some necessary meds were missing; the fourth-year student interested in anesthesiology substituted comparable ones. Every team member, naturally and without much discussion, created a role. This was an experience in teamwork that bound the group, became a touchstone that each would remember for years to come. Perhaps the foreign and meager surroundings summoned the best from each of us.

The baby's breathing became erratic, so Dr. Ed began to bag him, forced air into his lungs by compressing a small football-shaped-bag that was attached to a tiny mask. In the U.S. he would be intubated, a small tube inserted into his airway which would eventually be hooked up to a ventilator. But here with no ventilator, we could only continue bagging him for so long. Transportation to a Honduran hospital that was equipped to care for a baby this sick was a six-hour car ride through the mountains, and most of the road was unpaved. This baby was probably too ill to survive the trip. I led the discussion, "What is our endpoint here? I'm not sure it makes sense to intubate this baby."

"We can take turns bagging him."

"But we're talking six hours."

"You know what that road is like. We just did it by bus last week."

"But he looks a little better."

"Does the family have gas money? Money for the hospital?"

This was the poorest area of Honduras, just north of El Salvador and Nicaragua. During the 1980s, this part of the country had been a haven for anti-Sandinista contras, armed by the U.S., who fought the Marxist Nicaraguan government. The largely untillable fields possessed more hiding places between the rocky outcrops than valleys for growing crops. Landmines remained buried throughout the countryside, on both sides of the border, and occasionally injured the unlucky shepherd or cow.

"What does the family want?" I asked.

"Let's talk to Miguel."

Dr. Miguel, the local doctor, grew up in one of the larger Honduran cities and studied at the medical school in the capital, Tegucigalpa. He spoke excellent English. This end-of-life discussion was too complex for our ninth-grade translators. Besides, their lives and values were more like ours. Armed with their Ipods and cell phones, I doubted that they'd ever missed a meal or witnessed a death. They were first world meeting the third world in their own country.

In the dim hallway, just outside the room where we worked, Dr. Miguel spoke with the parents. He entered the room and told us that the parents wanted us to continue breathing for the baby until they could find the town's local lay minister to baptize their son. In this small town, the priest only came once a month to say Sunday mass, so a local woman ministered to the needs of the parish in his absence. Earlier in our stay, I'd attended the Sunday prayer service and received Communion from her.

After thirty long minutes, she arrived. A petite woman in her fifties, she had shoulder-length dark hair and not a strand of gray. Her pink blouse was neatly tucked into the waist of her navy knee-length straight skirt; she wore flip-flops. Calm but authoritative, she asked us to stop bagging the baby. We moved back from the exam table so she could perform the Baptism. She directed the mother to wrap the infant in his blanket and to hold him. She placed the father's hand on the baby's stomach. Reciting prayers, she dipped her fingers in the small glass jar of holy water she'd brought with her and made the sign of the cross over the baby. Then she flicked her wet fingers toward us. Droplets dampened my blue scrub top.

The mother sobbed as she clasped her infant, gently supporting his leg with the IV needle and tubing. The father grieved, muffled snivels into his shoulder, his dark, leathery hand on the baby's motionless body. Quietly the lay minister consoled them. Placing her calloused hands on both of their shoulders, she bowed her head and completed her prayers.

"Let's remove the IV line and take them to a private area where they can sit with the baby," Dr. Ed suggested.

Then we commiserated, "Should we stay with them?"

"What's culturally appropriate?"

"Let's ask."

Through a ninth-grade translator, we asked the parents what they wanted. They asked that staff sit with them, so Dr. Ed, a nurse, a medical student and the translator stayed. We moved them to a room that was used for clinic patients whom the doctor watched over night, since there was no hospital in town. A hospital bed and several chairs filled the space comfortably. The fluorescent tube in the ceiling hummed.

A few of us cleaned up the exam room where we had resuscitated the baby; morning clinic would start in nine hours. The rest of the team spread out on the clinic steps and talked. The clinic sat on a hill. The soccer game had ended hours earlier. Lights twinkled and cooking fires glowed inside the homes below. A pleasant coolness hung in the air. The ninth-grade translators, clustered on one corner of the stairs and chattered. How were they coping? One of the nurses checked in with them.

For the medical and nursing students and some of the family medicine residents, this was their introduction to international health where the rules and resources were different. At home "a code" was called and a shiny red cart filled with up-to-date supplies rolled into a well-lit room. Someone checked and restocked the cart after every use. There might be decisions about how much to do for a patient, but treatment for an infant like this would be clear-cut. He would be resuscitated, placed on a ventilator and admitted to the Neonatal Intensive Care Unit, heart monitor pads on his chest and an IV line inserted into a neck vein. One nurse would be assigned to care for him day and night.

The stark reality of what could be done in this clinic, in these mountains, hung before these future health care professionals. How could the skills they were diligently learning serve the people of rural Honduras? Here to help for a few weeks, what could they offer; could they make a difference?

Guilt about the excesses in our U.S. lives ballooned before us -- in the U.S. I was frustrated when my vacuum broke. But just down the hill in the two-room wooden shack with a dirt floor, a family of six settled in for the night. Did they have enough food for dinner? That morning we'd called on the grandfather to check and bandage the open wound on his leg. The students and translator who had accompanied me were appalled by the meager, but clean conditions in the shack. The floor was swept; dishes were drying on a linen towel on the wooden counter. The mother wore a spotless white apron.

As the evening progressed, there was a discussion about whether or not to give the family money. Generally this was discouraged, we had come to help — that was enough. The need was overwhelming. Once you gave to one person, how could you refuse another? And what kind of dynamic did giving money establish, where was the balance of power? What were you saying about the value of their work? What judgments were you passing on their standard of living?

But these circumstances seemed different and we took up a collection for funeral expenses. "The least we could do." At midnight, the watch continued. Realizing the team needed to go to bed in order to be rested for the next day's busy clinic, we divided into shifts so the on-call group would have a break.

The lay minister huddled in the room with the family and the on-call team. Some folks sat on the bed and additional chairs and stools had been pulled into the room. The infant lay swaddled in a blanket in his mother's arms. The group was silent, amplifying the hum of the lights and the volume of the infant's labored breathing; his face had a gray pallor. Minutes ticked by--this could last all night. About 2 a.m., as the nurse prepared to wake up the next shift, the infant stopped breathing for about twenty minutes. The lay minister performed last rights. Dr. Ed examined the infant and pronounced him dead. When the mother readjusted the baby's head, he sputtered and began breathing again.

All eyes in the room were now riveted on the infant. He took several slow breaths but intermittently quit breathing for five to ten minute intervals. Then, in the silence, he started to whimper. As he cried, his color changed from ashen to pink. The energy in the room shifted as if the sun had slipped from behind a cloud. The team whispered among themselves.

"What's going on?"

"Should we restart the IV?"

"This kid is supposed to be dead. He was septic when he came in."

"Did the antibiotics just kick in?"

"What do we tell the parents?"

The lay minister seemed to sense the confusion. She rose to her feet and through the translator talked about what had just happened. Her hands added emphasis. "This child has been reborn. This is not the child who was brought into the clinic sick and dying earlier this evening. This child, now baptized in the Lord, is a different child. Bless the Lord." When she stopped speaking, she made the sign of the cross, touching her forehead, chest and shoulders.

Then the father stood and explained that they wanted to take their son to a small hospital in El Salvador, just across the border, about a one-hour drive. He bowed slightly, "You have used your medicine. It was good medicine, and you have saved our son. You have done all that you can do. Now it is time for someone else to help him. Thank you for all of your hard work and care. *Gracias*"

Dr. Ed handed the father the funeral money, which they could use to purchase gas. The on-call team escorted the family out to their friend's car. The father roused the driver who was asleep in the back seat. The mother climbed into the front and the father handed her the swaddled infant. He slipped into the back behind the driver; the car door clicked shut. As they drove off, we watched the red taillights of the car wind down the hill and pondered what we have just witnessed.

The Pilgrim's Journey

In Mexico City at the shrine of Our Lady of Guadalupe, many worshipers crawl to the altar of Our Lady on their knees. The shrine of the Black Madonna is expansive. Elaborate gardens and the spacious plaza encircle the half-dozen older churches and the modern basilica. The trek for the worshipers stretches the equivalent of several city blocks: from the iron gate that separates the shrine from the vendors on the city street, across the worn stones of the plaza filled with tourists, then into the basilica that beckons with seven doorways. Inside, the space is open and airy and all aisles lead to the altar. Behind the altar, beneath the cross, suspended on a wooden pillar, enclosed in a golden brocaded frame and covered with glass, hangs their destination. The *tilma* (cloak) with the imprint of Our Lady of Guadalupe, the Black Madonna. Her dark skinned beauty is wrapped in a turquoise mantle and surrounded by a golden aura.

I sit in a wooden pew, half way back, after the eleven o'clock Mass concelebrated by six priests, and watch the penitents approach for the blessing. A *mujer* (woman) crawls cradling a swaddled baby with a bottle of milk in its mouth; three children wriggle behind, more game than devotion. One wears a neon-orange backpack out of which protrudes a magic wand — clear plastic with sparkles, a silver star and multi-colored ribbons dangling on the end. Their *abuela*, also on her knees, follows fingering a clear-beaded rosary. An older couple, arm in arm, walk behind her. Two teenage girls in provocative tank tops and mini-skirts hold hands and whisper to each other as they creep forward. Several dozen others approach, some walking, many on their knees.

My faith does not demand that I move toward the altar on my knees. But I am of the generation of Catholics that read the lives of the martyred saints as a child, was taught to venerate their tribulations and contritions. And I prayed for suffering, afflictions to purify my soul. During Lent, my family: Mom, Dad and six children, gave up their favorite treats. For most of my family it was chocolate; for me it was Lorna Doones.

Today I disagree with much of what the Catholic Church teaches: I believe in contraception; I believe that abortion should be an option; I believe any loving union whether same sex or male and female should be blessed; women should be allowed to be priests. Despite these differences, the Catholic ritual calls to me, quenches some thirst like a cold drink of water on a sticky summer day.

Through the years, my God has grown less judgmental and more benevolent. Call Him or Her the presence, higher power, or Spirit, with my God I strive to greet the world with compassion. At fifty, my practice is the blending of traditions: part Catholic, Native American, and Buddhist. God is most evident to me in nature: the spider web bejeweled with the morning's dew, sunrays beaming through the canopy of branches in a silent wood. I try to pay attention to each moment — mindfulness. My breath — inhale and exhale -- focuses me in my body and in the here and now. Breathe, I tell myself, whether I am with a patient, at the grocery checkout, or as I cut through the water in the pool during a workout. Breathe.

Situations that challenge me: the flat tire, the rude sales clerk, water in my basement, the losses and disappointments that constitute a life demand my attention and intention. The usual clichés apply: act as if, make lemonade out of the lemons, and find the "growth" opportunities. There are few bypasses in life; much of living is sweat, grit and attitude. I struggle to find my equilibrium and have learned to sit with and observe my frustration, anger and sadness. Eventually I recognize their transience. As a physician and scientist, I am most comfortable with reason, but sometimes life's circumstances push me beyond the rational to explore my helplessness, the many circumstances over which I have no control. A leap of faith is involved. I surrender to my breath and ask for grace and strength. I labor to identify the gifts in my life and pray in gratitude.

My eyes rest on the cloak of the Black Madonna behind the altar; I reflect on *milagros* (miracles). While working in the field in the fifteenth century, Our Lady appeared to Juan Diego and spoke to him in Nahuatl, his native language. She directed Juan to go to the archbishop and ask him to build a church on the rock where she was standing. Juan did as he was told, but the archbishop did not believe him. "Why would Our Lady appear to you, a poor peasant?" Disheartened, Juan returned to his work in the fields convinced that his vision of Our Lady must have been in his head. On December 12, the Virgin returned and instructed Juan to pick the roses that were miraculously blooming on the nearby hill that winter day and carry them to the archbishop as proof. Again, Juan did as he was told. When he opened his wrap to present the roses to the archbishop, Our Lady's picture was imprinted on the front of his cloak. Scientists and artists have examined the cloth and find the colors of the image embedded in the fibers. The cloak remains intact almost five centuries later.

I make the sign of the cross, touching the fingers of my right hand to my forehead, my heart, my right shoulder and then my left shoulder. This ritual familiar to me since childhood begins and ends a prayer. I reach for my black backpack behind the kneeler and scoot out of the pew moving into a less crowded aisle and toward the exit. Outside the basilica, the stones are uneven and worn; some are dark tones of gray and rust polished by centuries of prayerful steps. A few hold puddles from the rain earlier this morning. I wander around the corner into one of the older, smaller *igleseas* (churches). On a white-washed wall hangs a bulletin board covered in red felt framed with a ribbon of gold sequins. Near the top is a picture of a statue of Our Lady clothed in white lace. Pinned into the felt with straight pins are miniature legs, arms, hearts. Cows and horses. Human figures — some kneeling, some standing. Crafted from metal, all of these talismans of faith are available at the local gift shop. Tucked around them are photos, some in color and some black and white, corners curled: a plump toddler sucking his thumb; a thin boy in his crisply pressed school uniform; a young girl with her hair freshly combed, wearing a light blue dress with a lace collar, knobby kneed with patent leather shoes; a family posed on an asphalt street with mountains in the background; a couple arm in arm standing next to a Christmas tree. Folded notes scribbled on notebook paper are also pinned into the felt. Such evidence of faith, so much hope for divine intervention.

I've witnessed a handful of *Milagros*: At thirty, a close friend had a chest x-ray that showed a spot on his lung. His physician wanted to do a needle biopsy. My friend asked the physician to wait. Daily, my friend visualized its disappearance; saw the gray spot melt like butter on a piece of hot toast. One year later, his follow-up x-ray was clear.

A 59-year-old patient complained of pain in his pelvis. On exam, there was a palpable mass in his right lower abdomen. Tests confirmed an inoperable tumor, the worst kind. Refuting the odds, the patient and his family demanded treatment and underwent radiation therapy. With the support of his family, the patient reassessed his life, began regular exercise, and ate healthy foods. He joined a cancer support group and began meditation. He envisioned his good health. Several months and many tests later, the pathology confirmed only inflammation, no evidence of cancer.

There's been nothing so dramatic in my own life. Yet I have suffered desperation that has melted into clarity after a night of prayerful dreams. I've faced days with unmanageable challenges, and the critical face-off was implausibly removed. Plodded through twelve months of difficult events by searching for the wonders in the moments—the treble of a wren, the scent of phlox, the joke of a salesclerk and the smile of a child. Somewhere and somehow my backpack, heavy with tribulations grew lighter, acceptance took root and blossomed.

In *ciencia* (science) we are learning more about the mind-body interplay. Brain chemicals and immune modulators interact to affect health. We can "wish ourselves well" and "worry ourselves sick." We've all experienced getting sick when we are stressed or shortly after the completion of a big project. Studies show that the cells of the immune system are affected by psychosocial stressors or interventions that lead to health changes, especially with infections and wound healing. For example, volunteers who were inoculated with several different strains of the common cold viruses were more likely to get sick if their stress lasted more than a month. It took students longer to heal a wound in their mouths during exams than during vacation.

"The broken heart" is a reality. Depression and illnesses of the heart are common companions. One of five patients with coronary heart disease (blockage in the vessels of the heart) has depression, as does one of three patients with heart failure (the heart does not pump efficiently). Why? Perhaps the brain chemical changes that occur with depression make the heart more vulnerable. Or patients with depression may be less likely to take their heart medicines and make healthy choices such as exercising and eating the proper foods. Despite this growing knowledge, there is much more to learn.

As far back as 1955, scientists have studied the placebo effect. Give a patient a sugar pill or imitation therapy that they believe will help them and one out of three improve. Recent studies confirm the same, the placebo effect accounts for thirty percent. As a physician, I'll gladly take one out of three of my patients feeling better, because I provide hope.

I arrive at a side *capilla* (chapel). My eyes acclimate from the glare of the sunlight to the darkness inside. A hint of incense lingers and the fragrance of candle wax. It is quiet among the robed saints and votive candles. In Mexico the statues wear real clothes and often have human-like hair. I approach the shrine of Juan Diego and genuflect. The few pesos I drop in the metal box clatter as they hit the bottom. I touch a wooden match to a burning votive candle, light my own candle, make the sign of the cross, and whisper "Hail Mary full of grace . . ." These rituals, familiar to me since childhood, summon something deep within, a hunger to keep the faith.

Is there a difference between my faith and that of the penitents here? We both create room for the holy in our lives. We both have the capacity to trust something larger than ourselves. We move from the rational to the irrational without assurances. Perhaps some make this shift more easily than me.

It is simpler to care for patients who have a belief system that allows them to pray and hope. It provides a framework to approach and possibly accept the loss of control in their lives. To come to terms and make peace with their hardships: an injury that cripples a child, chronic pain, a terminal illness, death.

Research on the power of prayer is mixed. It is difficult research. How do you quantify prayer? What is the control--the prayer that is not prayer? To have a sound experiment it is necessary to have a group that receives the intervention and a group that does not (control) so the outcomes can be compared. The intervention group is prayed for; the control group receives words without intention. How do you evaluate intention?

I follow the stone stairs up the hill to the oldest chapel and with each step check the placement of my feet on the uneven steps. *Hay muchas escaleras.* (There are many stairs). I rest on the landings in between. On one families pay to have their children photographed. A placard with photos of posed children advertises the possibilities. The child is perched on a brightly painted wooden horse and some wear a sequin-studded yellow sombrero. Nearby a stand sells holy cards featuring the images of Juan Diego, the Black Madonna, or a cloak filled with roses; each has a Spanish prayer on the back.

From this vista I gaze over the roof tops of the churches: the modern basilica's smooth lines arch toward the sky, the old basilica cracked by the earthquake, the spires and domes of the smaller churches, all are crowned with crosses. Beyond extends the vast expanse of Mexico City, but here, the noise of the crowds and traffic is muted, the bells in the concrete-block bell tower a distant melodic jangle.

We with faith seek to accept life's events and challenges after struggling to lay some claim to what is essentially out of our control. We plead and hope for certain outcomes, then finally acquiesce to the hand of cards we are dealt. In the moments when I am metaphorically forced to my knees, I weep and gnash my teeth as well as anyone in the Bible. When weary I finally let go, surrender, and take that leap of faith. Only then I am able to focus on the moment and search for the hidden delights, the roses in the winter. Sometimes the roses bloom, perhaps a miracle; I am elated. If they freeze, then with belief in something greater than myself, larger than ourselves, there is an avenue for making sense of what seems essentially unfair. I cannot imagine coping without faith. My journey continues on to the top, and through my sandals I feel the scoop in the stones of these ancient stairs. Here is the worn path of all who have made this pilgrimage.

Dog Pals

Plain Jane is at least twenty years older than her housemates at the Women's Shelter, older than most of the staff too. Her home-permed bottle-brown hair frames her vacant expression, no smile, no frown. Her plump bottom crinkles the paper on the exam table in our small medical room off the back hall. She alternates between examining her hands that rest in the lap of her tan elastic-band slacks and making cautious eye contact with me as I question her. A gold band and small diamond ring encircle her left fourth finger.

She is the third patient on my schedule. The medical students, first and second years, are behind on triaging, so I have time to talk with her. The students and I provide medical services to the moms and kids at the local shelter every Tuesday. It is a win-win for all: free services for shelter residents; a chance for me to learn more about intimate-partner abuse, my research interest; and the opportunity for the students to practice their newly acquired interview and examination skills.

Jane responds with one- or two-word answers. I am working hard to understand why she wanted to be seen, but something shifts when I ask her about her marriage.

"He yelled at me thirty of our thirty-eight years," she says, her expression deadpan. She extends her hand with the rings, then clenches the fingers to her palm. "Hit me at least forty times with his hand. Lot of power in his fist. You can't imagine."

"I'm sure I can't," I reply, reflecting on what *loved ones* do to each other in the privacy of the home.

"If only he'd stop yellin'," she continues. Her face does not convey her obvious frustration. She should play poker.

"In fact, the woman who answered the crisis line could hear him shoutin'. Told me I'd be safer in another city. Better to come to the big city." She shakes her head, her tight curls bobbing. "Quite a temper. Called me every name in the book."

I review her long list of pills: blood pressure, cholesterol, diabetes, anxiety, sleep, pain and depression. No allergies. Warming the stethoscope between my hands, I ask her about chest pain, breathing trouble, arthritis. I ramble off the usual list.

She affirms most of the above. I sigh to myself, not surprised. I reflect on how she's honed the emptiness, the passivity, no reaction. Did it limit the abuse? Did he hit her more or less if she cried? Or was it her defense, you can't really get to me, can't hurt me, can't damage me. Instead, her body and heart are broken.

I lift her plaid blouse and listen to her heart and lungs, feel her thick neck for masses and check her ankles for swelling, then perch on my stool to listen some more. "Did you ever talk with your doctor about the abuse?" I ask.

Jane nods, the wrinkles of her chin stretch and contract like an accordion. "My last visit I told doctor that my husban' was gettin' kind a rough. He told me to have him make an appointment with him. Wasn't 'bout to do that. A sure way to get my head knocked off."

Baffled at a colleague's apparent lack of knowledge, I mull over the amount of training work to do. For almost twenty years the American Medical Association has encouraged physicians to ask about intimate partner violence, less than ten percent do, like learning to inquire about cigarettes thirty or forty years ago. "What brought you here?" I ask.

Her shoulders quiver, her fingers stroke her forehead, and tears pool in her eyes, puddle in a wrinkle, then spill over like a miniature waterfall. After a deep exhale, she whispers, "My dogs." Then her shoulders shudder and she sobs, unable to continue.

I am puzzled, hand her a box of tissues and readjust myself on the stool. I am afraid to touch her, don't want to invade her boundaries. Still no medical students knock; I have time for this.

Her weeping subsides to whimpers and she dabs at her eyes, no mascara smudges. She blows her nose, a honking sound. With her composure regained, she continues. "They were old, but they were my babies." She describes the one who slept at her feet, cuddling against her. The other lay on the rug at the side of her bed, a sentinel. "Gettin' old, nothin' fancy, just mutts, but my babies." She spoke about her dogs as one would a lover, a dear friend.

I think about my own dog, Tobi, and his unconditional love. I could yell at him in the morning, but he'd greet me in the evening with unabated enthusiasm and charm. He stretched out on the floor with this front paws crossed and his right ear perpetually cocked. I was forever charmed by his adoring green eyes.

"When I got up at night to go to the bathroom, they followed me."

I often sang *Me and My Shadow* to my dog--*walking down the avenue* . . .

"When he yelled at me they stood right next to me. 'Bout a month ago he told me to git rid of 'em. Jealous maybe." She is silent, staring off into the corner of the room. "I started tryin' to find a home for 'em. But who wanted two old fogies, one had a stroke, the other arthritis . . . didn't always make it out the door in time to pee . . ."

I think of my own dog, who stopped eating when my ex and I split before the divorce. After I found a place that would accommodate a dog, Tobi took interest in his food again, but not until he was with me.

Jane is mumbling now. I lean close to hear her words. "Shortly before I came here he took both dogs without tellin' me and had 'em put to sleep. I know they were old . . ." The tears return.

I choke back my own tears, feeling her pain and grief, my own recent loss. A month ago Tobi was killed on the highway a mile from my home. I am not sure what he was doing out there, probably scavenging, a survival skill he'd acquired early in life (he was a rescue). A neighbor called to tell me she thought it was mine, a black and white dog hit that morning on her way to work. He was missing the night before, and I was afraid, imagining the worst. I recovered his cold, stiff body at the intersection at the end of the workday. It was dusk, a bone-chilling drizzle. Thrusting his rigid body into the trunk of my car, I sobbed. When the ground thawed, I gave him a proper burial.

I struggle to keep my composure. A tap at the door jars me from contemplating our mutual losses, the dog pals killed, the darkness of the act that precipitated her leaving after thirty-eight years. I respond to the knock, a moment to compose myself, and tell the students that I'll be done in a few minutes.

Jane opens her purse, pulls out her wallet and hands me a picture of her two, red felt bows around their necks, obviously a Christmas shot. "Trixy and Mabel," she croons, a proud mama. Her tears under control, she tells me that when she cried about the loss of the dogs, he hit her in the shoulder. He never had a name, just "he." "He said I cared more for them, than him."

"They treated you better," I say, angry at him and sad for her, and still struggling to keep a professional demeanor. Over the years I'd learned that it was okay to cry with patients, a way to show empathy. Besides once the faucet started dripping, it was hard to shut it off.

She is weeping as well, nodding in agreement. "They treated me like a queen."

I hand her a tissue, take one myself and whisper, "I'm sorry this happened." Frustrated by the inadequacy of the words and caught in the web of my own painful memories, I reach for her hand. She clutches my hand like a small child holds on to mama. When her tears subside, I ask her if she dreams about her dogs, remembering my own dream. Sometimes in the middle of the night I can feel Tobi licking my face, would swear that my skin was damp from his moist rough tongue.

Jane sniffles and nods, slowly telling me about her dream. "The dog with the stroke, Trixy, is curled next to me." She says that she is afraid to pet Trixy, thinking she might be dead. But when she does, Trixy is warm with life and licks her hand.

Another rap at the door summons me back to the tasks at hand. I thank Jane for sharing her dog pals with me and scribble prescriptions for the medications she needs. As much as I want to, I have no power to change Jane's life, make these next weeks and months easier as she proceeds with divorce.

Or she might decide that that route is too hard; she's lived with the abuse for so long, she'll put up with it until the end, when one of them dies. I cannot stop her from returning to her husband. But here for this moment, we connected over our shared loss. Perhaps that in itself is healing; I know it is for me.

Meeting Daniel

An olive skinned boy with familiar doe-like eyes and close-cropped hair perches on the stool in the corner of the exam room. Daniel is my six-year-old patient for a well-child check, the third of the morning at the community clinic. He concentrates on his dirty tennis shoes, but glances up when I enter the room. A generously proportioned African-American woman accompanies him: his mom, I wonder. I introduce myself.

"He's been with me for a month," she says. "I don't know much about him."

Not his mom: foster care. I wonder about his story.

"But I think he has had trouble with asthma," she continues. "He has an inhaler, but no problems since he's been with me." She pulls folded papers from her large black purse.

"Have you cared for children with asthma?" I ask.

She nods. Daniel sits silently and continues to examine his sneakers. We talk about potential asthma triggers and the problem cough. The papers she has with her don't say much about his past medical history, only that he has no allergies. Has he been hospitalized for asthma? Been to the emergency department? Had trouble with his ears, PE tubes, Tonsils out? She can't answer my questions, and Daniel adds nothing. I vent my frustration with a silent exhale; it's not their fault.

Quiet and obedient Daniel responds to my questions. School— getting used to a new place. Wetting the bed—no. His favorite food--pizza. I ask him to climb up on the exam table; he shows good coordination. I peer in his ears with the otoscope; an old PE tube sits in the right canal. As I examine him and watch his reticent responses, I become convinced that I've inspected him before. "You've seen me before?" I watch his sad, knowing eyes.

He shrugs, raises his eyebrows, and picks at the paper on the exam table.

I listen to his heart and lungs and ask him to blow my finger like he's blowing a candle. He complies. He knows the routine.

"No wheezes today." I compliment Daniel and ask Foster Mom how things are going at home.

"They reported problems, but he's well-behaved for me. Plays well with my grandsons." Her broad lips curve up as she gazes at Daniel.

How many children has she nurtured? Probably dozens. I concentrate on Daniel. "Have you been in many foster homes?"

"Lots." He stares at his tennis shoes, swinging them against the exam table. A soft bop, bop, bop . . . They close with a Velcro strap.

"Do you know what's going on with his mom?"

"Substance abuse and mental problems," Foster Mom murmurs.

Finishing his examination, I check genitals (circumcised) and talk about good touch and bad touch. I ask him to stand on the linoleum floor and touch his toes, and I check his spine for straightness. Then, I instruct him to imitate me: stand on his right foot and then his left. He follows. He imitates my one-foot-in-front-of-the-other tight rope walk. There is both boredom and comfort in the routine, the third time I'd performed the exam that morning. If my attitude is right, and my focus is on the child, it becomes a prayer, the "ritual of the well-child check."

Neurons and synapses fire and connect in my brain. "Daniel, I know where I met you. Did you and your mom live at the shelter — the big old brick house?"

He stares blankly, and then his expression shifts, like the rising sun slipping into view between a fracture in the clouds. His eyes widen. "The one with the winding stairs?"

I nod and remember his mother. She had the same doe-like eyes; she was small-framed and spoke English with a subtle Mexican accent, rolling her *r*s. Daniel was her pride and joy, and she kept detailed records in a pocketsize, spiral blue notebook. On at least two occasions, she'd brought him to the weekly clinic at the local battered women's shelter. Daniel and his mother had stayed at the shelter for a month, left, and returned several months later, only six months ago. I never saw her as a patient, so I didn't know her story, only that she was committed to Daniel and meticulous about Daniel's ear infections and asthma. She'd arranged follow-up for him at the children's hospital clinic when they moved out of the shelter.

What had intervened in her mothering? Did she return to the abuser, her boyfriend or Daniel's dad, and as a result children's services deemed her an unfit mother, failure to protect Daniel? Did she have an alcohol or drug problem and start using again? Had she run out of her anti-depressant or anti-anxiety meds and become unstable, another reason to deem her unfit? Had the system failed her?

I have worked with the system long enough to know its imperfections. Everyone is well intentioned, but moms and kids fall through the cracks, lose health insurance and cannot afford medications despite my attempts to provide samples. They return to abusers because they cannot afford to live on their own or they want fathers for their kids. This complexity and uncertainty are facts of life.

Daniel stands between his foster mom and me. I've taken his place on the stool. He examines his sneakers again. I wish the answers were woven in the stitching. My heart trembles as if a string is plucked. For a moment, I want to take him home, give him stability. I want to tell him that he has a dedicated mom who adores him, and wants the best for him, struggles to care for him. I want to see him in five years, ten years, to remind him of this. If only I could wave a magic wand and assure him that his life will turn around -- stable home, school, the love of healthy parents. I want to promise him that he will not grow up to be a drug addict, an abuser or repeat the patterns of his folks. Unfortunately, I cannot give him any guarantees; there is no insurance to protect him from these possibilities. At this moment, I can only assure Foster Mom and Daniel that today he is a healthy six-year-old, and we will give him his kindergarten shots.

Denial: Titrating the Truth

As a medical student, I saw denial as a bad thing. I recall an attending physician's anger at a patient's family who would not admit that their father, my patient, was dying from cancer. Then during residency, there was Jean, an alcoholic, who could not see her problem. She only had a "little" drink of whiskey every night.

"How much?" I'd asked.

The tips of her fingers, with long painted red nails, moved apart four inches.

"A water glass?" I asked.

Jean nodded.

I never did convince her that her little drink was a problem.

***

Rosemary had many reasons to fight for her life. Her busy daughter managed the modern version of the old general store in our small community of 3000. Rosemary took care of the household, played taxi driver for her preteen granddaughter and was the emotional stalwart in the family. She also loved golf.

Rosemary had a hard time saying "cancer." Her smoker's laugh rumbled from deep in her pelvis, about the same location where her rectal tumor grew, now unresponsive to a second round of chemo. A Twins baseball cap concealed her thinning hair and softened the sharp features of her emaciated face. She greeted me: "Hi Doc, I don't want to take up your time." That's how she started most of our visits.

Eighteen months earlier, she had complained of fatigue. Searching for the cause, I checked her hemoglobin. When the lab report read eight (normal is closer to 12, even in a seventy year old woman), I suspected a cancer somewhere in her colon. A colonoscopy detected the tumor and she soldiered through surgery and chemotherapy. After a year of remission, the cancer returned and she submitted to a second round of chemo. Its failure was signaled by a nodule, about the size of a nickel, which grew on her back. I fingered the lesion and struggled to keep my voice steady as I explained how the cancer cells had moved into her lymph system and traveled throughout her body.

The nature of our visits changed. We now focused on managing her pain, an ache deep in her groin. "Take the pain medicine on a regular basis, mornings and evenings, so the pain doesn't get ahead of you."

"But I don't want to be addicted," she said. "And it makes me so tired." That day she'd forgotten her baseball cap. Her scalp resembled that of a baby's head sprouting a few strands of gray fuzz.

"We can deal with tired. Let's get the pain under control." I told her about Ritalin, the prescription version of speed, which would help her appetite and give her some pep.

Her blue-gray eyes widened as she cackled, "Me taking speed." She declined that, but agreed to take her pain medicine on a schedule. Then there was the nausea, which made it hard to eat, but a new medicine would address that. "I feel like a pharmacy, so many pills," she complained.

When she returned a week later, she'd lost three more pounds and her cheek bones carved even deeper hollows in her pale face. She reported feeling full after two spoonfuls of food. The pain still bothered her, and she had no energy to play golf.

"I have a question," she said and reached for my pen and paper. She scrawled, "Is it cancer pain" followed by a big question mark.

I nodded.

Tears filled her eyes. "I was hoping it was arthritis."

I thought she knew this. I touched her dry and warm hand. Where should I start? Our conversation would take time, but at this point, time was all I had to offer Rosemary; my other patients would have to wait.

Denial is powerful. Denial is protective. Rosemary took in what she was able to hear; like her food, she consumed a few tablespoons of truth at a time. Once she digested that, she was ready for a little more. A few weeks earlier, I had suggested hospice. She completed the intake interview, but fired the hospice nurse after her first visit, complaining that she was too pushy. "I'm just not that sick," Rosemary told me.

I wanted Rosemary to enroll because it was the most expedient way to improve her comfort. Hospice would manage her pain and Rosemary's family would benefit from the additional support. I chewed my lip, disappointed, when hospice services told me that she didn't want them to return. But I respected Rosemary's wishes.

A few weeks later, she had lost even more weight. I suggested hospice again. This time she was ready. When the hospice nurse returned, she ignored the earlier awkward interactions, tended to Rosemary's comfort and supported her family. I learned to titrate the information I gave her and to respect her timeline. Her body was doing things beyond her control — new growths, fatigue, nausea and pain -- and Rosemary desperately wanted to control what she could.

***

When I visited Nicaragua in January, denial appeared in a dramatic form. For the last four Januarys, I have volunteered with a nonprofit that has worked in a northern community for over fifteen years. After a sweltering and busy day in clinic, several colleagues and I climbed the hill through the poorest neighborhood to sip cold beers on the patio of the town's nicest hotel. Suddenly Philippe, age nineteen, walked toward us. Since we had arrived, a rumor had circulated that his sixteen-year-old brother was in prison for murder. I had been anxious to talk with Philippe. I hugged him.

The nonprofit's bus rolled into the community four times a year and Philippe and his brother, Antonio, had always greeted us at the hotel where we stayed. During my first year, we had played Sudoku every night after dinner. I practiced my Spanish; they practiced their English and we shared the common language of numbers. They assisted with the construction crew's projects until the laws changed and child labor became a concern. We paid them to polish our shoes and purchased their hand-woven bracelets or the other trinkets they sold.

Several of the long-time volunteers had "adopted" the two boys. The head of construction paid for their English lessons, another set up an account to pay for their schooling. These "benefactors" occasionally received additional requests--money for a new bed for mama, a new roof and additional schoolbooks.

A serious and driven young man, Philippe had applied to medical school but did not get in. Now he took courses at the local college. Last year, Antonio, the charming and cuter kid brother, had blossomed into a handsome teen.

That afternoon on the patio, peacocks squawked in the distance. Our beers and cokes sweated as did I when Philippe told us his brother had been falsely accused of murder. In fact, he said, "Antonio was in bed with me. He'd gone to church and then come home."

Others in the town told a different story: Over the last six months, Antonio had gotten into drugs and pimping. A man had not paid for his time with a prostitute, so Antonio had settled the debt with his machete. Which story was true? Of course, I wanted to believe Philippe, but too many reliable locals told us that Antonio had changed and was probably guilty.

Philippe needed $1000 to hire a lawyer for his brother. "Can you help me?" he sobbed. The news shocked all of us. What was the truth? How could Philippe be in denial about his brother committing a murder? Was Philippe conning us for more money? Could we turn our backs on Philippe? Could I turn my back on a four-year relationship during this time of great need? I was a rich American; I did not want to be an ugly American, but I did not want to support Philippe's illusion. And I did not want to be taken advantage of. Between the haves in America and the have-nots of Nicaragua, there would always be requests for money. How should we respond? How should I respond?

I deliberated and prayed. As the morning light filtered through the curtains, I pulled on my running shoes and headed outside. The golden sun inched above the mountains burning through the mist that hovered over the tobacco fields. The air hung fresh. I sorted through my options: Philippe was asking with the best intentions. Because of our four-year relationship, I trusted that his belief and request were sincere, that he wanted to help his brother, that he was not conning me. For him, the truth about his brother was too awful to swallow. Despite the heinous act, in this family-first culture, he had a responsibility to his brother. How could I support Philippe, but not play into his denial?

I have come to see denial as curious, how the mind protects us from what we are unable to bear. Negotiating around denial can be irritating and cumbersome. But if I am a healer, if I want to help, then I must figure out how to maintain a connection with the patient or the family despite their denial. The truth may be obvious to me, but the path to understanding for the patient or the family is less clear. I have to figure out how to support them.

As a family doctor, I deal with patients' denial in order to better manage a variety of chronic conditions -- diabetes, heart disease, depression. I've become deft at moving in sideways, to gently poke at the denial and resistance, often with humor, as I search for a connection and build the trust to maneuver forward. As a doctor, my job is to partner with the patient on the journey, to try to help manage what seems foreign and impossible.

Denial is part of life. We all struggle with the truth that ultimately there is much over which we have no control.

With Rosemary, we revisited the management of her illness until her fate grew unavoidably clear. Until she came to terms with her diagnosis, she suffered more than I wanted her to and her family struggled to care for her. I had to manage my own inability to control her choices.

As a physician, I have the privilege of sitting on the sidelines of life and observing the human struggle, watching others as they face the wonder and terror of being. This privileged view, seeing how patients grapple with the challenges life hands them, gives me insight into my own struggles.

With my own challenges, I have learned to honor my process. I examine my feelings — discomfort, anger, sadness. As with patients, I sit though the inevitable cycles -- the denial, the acceptance, the fear, and hope for grace. Sometimes it arrives. To be present and give my full attention to my patients and to myself is really all I can do.

Before I left Nicaragua, I told Philippe that I could not give him money for a lawyer, but *"usted esta hermano bueno, you are a good* brother." I lectured him on the importance of not losing site of his own goals. Philippe's "family first" culture might pressure him to sacrifice his education and his future for his brother's legal fees. I handed him $20 to cover the cost of several one-hour bus trips and food to visit his brother in prison. Twenty was a pittance compared to the amount he requested, but it was a gesture toward helping him, a sideways approach to his request.

***

Postscript: The next year, I learned that Antonio had been released from prison because there was not enough evidence to convict him. Locals still believed that he was guilty, but told us that the parties involved would not harm him.

Expectations, Disappointments and Surprises: The Rough Waters of Narcotic Dependence

Prescribing controlled substances is a dreaded duty for most physicians I cannot live up to patients' expectations and demands, and invariably I disappoint.

"You'll be a good doctor for her," the internist said handing me a manila envelope. "She wants a woman." I flipped through the papers; her diagnoses read--Chronic jaw pain, Headaches, Fibromyalgia with at least five surgeries, Depression, Narcotic dependence, Narcotic abuse. Susan was referred to me because I had the reputation of "compassionate doctor," one willing to take the time to work with "challenging" patients, but when I reviewed her hospital discharge, I wanted to scream, "No please not me, find someone else." Susan's medication staircase read: Codeine, Vicodin, Morphine, Percocet, Dilaudid.

With her array of problems and narcotic use, she would be a "heart sink" patient -- when her name appeared on my phone log or schedule, my heart would race and pound. I'd calm myself with slow deep breaths, as if on the high dive, then I'd take the plunge, tap on the wooden door, turn the metal knob and enter the room wearing my empathy.

Susan shoved an envelope of medical records at me, this pack two inches thick. "Please review these. The other doctors didn't bother." Her voice was high and childlike. Her eyes locked with mine for an uncomfortable second and I swallowed hard at her expectations of me.

She was middle-aged, slightly overweight, with a faint smell of perfume. Her pale skin appeared even whiter in contrast to her dark, shoulder-length hair. She settled into the plastic chair, smoothed her navy skirt over her knees, and fingered the cuffs of her yellow blouse.

Turning the computer screen toward her, my hand on the mouse, I clicked "Patient History" and then invited her to review the diagnoses I'd compiled from my earlier review of her hospitalization summary.

She scanned the list. "Narcotic dependence and abuse." Her voice jumped an octave and her spine stiffened. "I only do what doctors tell me."

Her observation, I told myself. She had no insight into her addiction. I took a breath, and then suggested that we review the rest of her history. Susan had moved to Minnesota from the South in search of a more wholesome place to raise her children. Physicians at another Minnesota clinic had informed her that Minnesota doctors would be reluctant to prescribe narcotics for someone her age. She promptly stopped all her meds and was hospitalized for severe vomiting and diarrhea, withdrawal symptoms from the abrupt discontinuation of narcotics. On discharge, she was given some Percocet and an appointment with a pain clinic.

"How many Percocet do you take a day?" I asked.

"Two," she said.

"And on a bad day?"

She paused, adjusted her glasses, and glanced at the floor, "Well, maybe five . . . "

"When was the last time you had a bad day?" I asked.

"A . . . Monday was kind of tough," she drawled, her southern accent was pronounced as she reached for a tissue.

"How many did you take then?" I persisted, pushing the box closer to her.

"Well, two in the morning and two in the afternoon and maybe two to help me sleep."

"How do you sleep?"

She sighed. "Lousy."

I breathed deeply to ground myself and summoned more empathy; Susan's pain was real. If we were going to form a therapeutic relationship, I had to gain her trust. I also had to understand the context of her life. I asked about her support system. Her husband was gone from home for months at a time. Essentially, she was raising two young children and one teen on her own. The teenager, a girl, tested her constantly. She'd had some truancy and did not obey the limits her mother set.

Susan had married her high school sweetheart. "He's so wonderful," she gushed. "The love of my life" she told me as her pupils dilated and took on that glassy haze of someone in love. She paused then continued, "It's wonderful when he's home. The oldest wouldn't think of disobeying him."

I leveled my tone and asked about the challenges when Susan's husband returned home. "Switching from single- to co-parenting can be tough," I said.

Susan stared at the yellow Espadrilles on her feet. "At times he drinks to relax."

I'd found the soft spot in this southern peach. Mustering compassion, I followed Susan's hint, "How does he act then?"

She glanced past me and stared toward the floor again. "I stay out of his way." Running her hand through her black hair, she told me that her parents were alcoholics. "I know when to take the kids and go shopping, go visit a friend . . ."

There was no admission about needing to numb herself, but she had the classic signs of drug dependence: pain that required increasing amounts of narcotics and the onset of violent illness when she stopped them. The source of her pain could not be identified by tests. Actual pain, from heartache and disappointment, transmuted to the body. I tried to explain this.

Again, she fixed on a point beyond me, her arms folded against her breasts, her lips pursed.

I refilled all of Susan's non-narcotics. At two pills a day, she had enough Percocet to last until her pain clinic appointment in two weeks, so she wouldn't go through withdrawal again. I pointed this out, offered my hand, which she clasped in both of hers and thanked me for being kind. We agreed that she would return to see me after her visit with the pain specialist. She left the clinic with my letter for the pain specialist that listed her medical diagnoses, including narcotic dependence and abuse, current medications, allergies, and the vitals from the day's visit.

Later that day I heard from the office manager that Susan had called from home furious that my letter to the pain specialist said that she was both narcotic dependent and an abuser.

The skilled manager had asked Susan to write a letter documenting her concerns. The letter would become part of her medical record. I was grateful that I didn't have to call her back.

As I completed my charting for the day, I second-guessed my conclusions and reviewed her previous records — had I labeled her unfairly? Notes from nurses and physicians indicated increasing demands for narcotics, concerns about lost medications and early prescription refills, the usual signs of abuse. "Denial is part of the illness," I told the manager. "The abuse diagnosis stands. I'll discuss it with her when she returns for her follow-up appointment."

She never did.

I was not the compassionate doctor she was hoping to meet. Some doctors brush off the anger of the narcotic dependent patient who doesn't get what they want — labeling the patient a jerk and leaving it at that. Other physicians give in and have the reputation of being easy. Some refuse to prescribe narcotics and hence, avoid the messy interactions. Sometimes the patient's manipulation takes the form of a sob story and I feel like an ass until I hear the familiar hints, and finally the request that confirms my suspicion. "I'm allergic to ibuprofen. Tylenol #3 doesn't really work, but Vicodin does." At times the asking is more direct. "I've moved and the lifting killed my back. Can I have some Percocet?"

These interactions require me to be thick skinned. They never make me feel good about my work, and the interactions feel messy and unsettling. I've told myself that narcotic dependant patients need caring doctors, too, especially in a small town. I've tried to be compassionate, but firm.

Like Susan, Eleanor wanted a primary care doctor to prescribe her narcotics. I met her after her pain clinic consultations for chronic headaches and neck pain. We agreed to the recommended narcotic schedule, then reviewed and signed a contract. She agreed to get narcotics from our clinic only and from one pharmacy. She could not ask for more, even if she lost her medications, and we'd obtain periodic urine screens.

I learned from the nurses that ten years earlier she'd come to the clinic weekly for a Demerol shot. With time, she admitted to leaving an abusive marriage. Now, her six children were grown.

Sometimes the pain was bad and Eleanor took extra pills, asking me for more. I declined. We discussed other ways to manage the pain — taking walks, using ice, distraction, and prayer. "The pain won't kill you," I said. "Your body craves more medicine. You can't give in to the craving." She lost a job, which exacerbated her depression. We adjusted her antidepressants. Eleanor started seeing a therapist. She volunteered at the Food Shelf, walked routinely, and tried to enjoy her grandchildren. After increased cravings, she visited the pain clinic again and they suggested either starting a new medication for which we would need to get a prior authorization or decreasing her dose for the month. Eleanor chose the latter; it was a hard month, but she managed.

One day, fed up with her reliance on her pain medications, Eleanor flushed them down the toilet. The nausea, abdominal cramps and sweats of withdrawal made for a miserable time. She came to see me realizing she should not have discarded her meds and hoping that I'd prescribe additional ones.

I said no. "I am sorry about what you've gone through and what's ahead. But I can't violate our contract." We discussed the other ways she could distract herself.

Eleanor stared at her lap and clutched her purse. Sweat beaded on her temples.

My stethoscope lay heavy against my neck. I realized the power I had as a physician, the power to make decisions about a patient's life and comfort, about a patient's addiction. With the license came obligations to myself and the patient.

Eleanor returned a month later. She wore carefully applied makeup and smelled of soap; she looked more put together than then at our last visit. I asked her how she had done.

"It was hard." And then — "It was a particularly bad day. I was praying, trying to ignore the pain, trying to remember what you told me — that the pain wouldn't kill me. It's just a nuisance." She glanced toward me. "I don't know if you'll understand this, but I felt God's presence. The world opened and a warm light surrounded me. I knew I would be okay. He reassured me that I would have peace. I could deal with my pain. I felt a comfort I've never felt before. My dad's a minister so I told him about it. He said it was a spiritual experience."

I stopped typing on the computer key pad. We sat in silence each of us thankful for her experience. Her success was a gift for me, a confirmation that my "tough love," had been the right response. She'd been shown that there was something beyond the medications.

With narcotics dependent patients, I often feel like a parent managing a teen -- the same cantankerous tension. I had felt bad about saying no, knowing the miserable week she'd have, but I had to. My quandary was not about being liked by Eleanor, but doing what I thought served her best.

Eleanor's experience was a gift for her and a gift for me, an affirmation. My limit setting had yielded an unexpected surprise and affirmation for both of us. With Susan, I was not so lucky. Both encounters remind me that I don't have complete control of the relationship or the outcome. My responsibility is to do my part as honestly and compassionately as I can.

Living and Dying Well

Crunch. Her ribs cracked as I thrust my palms down on her bird-like chest.

Crunch. Press. Press. Try to restart her heart.

She was eighty-five years old, for heaven's sake. Her skin was like tissue paper stretched over bones. She looked so frail in her hospital bed, the antiseptic smell swirling around us. It seemed cruel, inhumane. But we didn't have a code status, so my resident directed me to start CPR. And I broke her ribs. Torture. That is what it was, torture — for her and me. I did not want to do CPR; couldn't we just let her die peacefully? This was not the way to end a long life. But what could we do with a little old lady "found down" — collapsed on her back porch and discovered by a neighbor — with no identified family? It just wasn't right. But we kept at it until my resident called the code.

Jane Hamilton was officially dead.

Dying is part of doctoring. As a young doctor completing a family medicine residency at the county hospital in St. Paul, Minnesota, I encountered patients like Jane and agonized about the experiences. It was the mid-1980s, and policies about dying and resuscitation were still being established. Even with the technological capabilities in medicine at that time, I needed to understand more than I'd learned in medical school about the dying process. Although we have come a long way, medical training still focuses on how to save lives, and physicians struggle with knowing how to help patients have a peaceful death. Both DNR (Do Not

Resuscitate) orders and advanced directives are commonplace, but unfortunately many physicians don't make full use of them.

Dr. Elizabeth Kubler-Ross's groundbreaking book, *On Death and Dying*, first published in 1969, synthesized the experience of two hundred terminally ill patients at the University of Chicago. Although her work was considered "soft science" because she only did interviews, she initiated a national discussion about a respectful end to life. Physicians began to talk with their patients who had terminal illnesses, like cancer, about whether or not they wanted CPR at the end of their lives. Since being established and distributed throughout the U.S. in the 1960s, CPR had become the standard of care to perform if a patient's heart stopped beating. But sometimes this seemed to prolong a patient's agony, especially in a patient with an illness like cancer. About the same time, the hospice movement, which started in the United Kingdom, reached the U.S. After the success of her book, Kubler-Ross started her own healing center and conducted workshops for both health professionals and patients around the world.

Following the death of Jane Hamilton, on the advice of a colleague and mentor, I signed up for Kubler-Ross's week-long workshop on death and dying. After a busy day in clinic, I caught an evening flight and arrived in Arizona. The workshop was held at a chemical dependency treatment complex on the outskirts of Tucson, where the residents of the center shared their ranch-style dining and conference rooms with the workshop attendees. As I waited for the front desk attendant to locate a bed for me, I shed the layers of clothing required in Minnesota's frigid temperatures — down jacket, woolen scarf, and gloves — and breathed in sage and creosote, fragrances so different from those of home.

Inside my cottage seven roommates slept in single beds; the open bed in the center of the room left for me. (I learned later that three other women had come and gone from that bed before I finally claimed it at midnight). I was so tired, having spent most of the prior night admitting patients to the hospital in Minnesota, and now the full force of my exhaustion hit me. I was relieved to leave my residency and all my patient duties thirteen hundred miles away. I unpacked my suitcase and slipped into my flannel nightgown. The room felt cramped. Someone snored. Another roommate mumbled in her sleep. Near the bathroom lay a woman, bald, with the faint sour scent of sickness, probably some type of cancer. I was surprised to see someone so ill, but would learn later that Kubler-Ross encouraged patients and health professionals to attend the same workshops. Soon, I too snuggled under my covers and fell asleep.

The words *I can't breathe* jolted me awake. I sat up, still in doctor mode, now always in doctor mode. The clock flashed 1 a.m. I heard shouts coming from the beds near the bathroom. Someone had turned on the bathroom light. I jumped out of bed, the floor cold on my bare feet.

"I can't breathe," the bald woman panted. She had the chipmunk cheeks often caused by the medication prednisone. Propped up against pillows, she gasped for air, her hands thrashing. Her face was red like a radish with a fine sheen of sweat. "Help me, help me . . . ," she choked.

I stared at her from my position at the foot of her bed. I did not know her, did not know her medical history, but I guessed chemotherapy had caused her baldness. A zip lock bag filled with pill bottles sat on her bedside table. A folded wheelchair leaned against the wall. The woman who had been in the next bed spoke with her and tried to calm her.

I needed to do something; after all I was a doctor. I stumbled to her side and blurted, "How can I help? I'm a doctor." Her arm was clammy and sticky, like a fish.

But the bald woman was not consoled. "I can't breathe. I can't breathe. Help me. Help . . . "

My red flannel provided no protection from her panic.

My other roommates were now out of their beds, all the lights in the room turned on. We crowded around the bed like bees hovering around a hive.

"Does she have oxygen?" I asked.

"There's a physician somewhere at the retreat center," another said. "He knows something about her. I'll find him." She threw on her coat, slipped into clogs, and sprinted out the door.

The bald woman continued to thrash and cry, her face now purple. I offered water, rummaged through her pills. Damn, I thought I'd left these situations back in Minnesota. I had come to the workshop for some self-care and reflection, and now only hours after my arrival I was called into action. I resented it and at the same time felt helpless, no tools, no information.

Gasp. Pant. Thrash. Sheets twisted and mashed.

The bungalow's door swung open, and the roommate returned with a man dressed in jeans and a plaid shirt cradling an oxygen tank in his arms like an infant. He took charge. "Her name is Chloe. She has metastatic breast cancer," he said. "I've called the medics." He set the tank next to the bed and slipped a plastic mask over her face.

I stuttered that I was a doctor and could help. I had to say it twice. When he finally heard me, he smiled and directed me to wipe her forehead with a cold cloth.

I could do that. I hurried to the sink in the bathroom and returned with a cold washcloth.

Two medics burst through the door and immediately went to work. Dressed in navy blue uniforms, one carried a cardiac monitor, the other a case of medications and supplies. I squeezed against the wall to make room for them. One checked for a pulse, then wrapped the blood pressure cuff around Chloe's arm. The other unbuttoned her nightshirt, stuck pads on her chest and clipped wires to the cardiac monitor.

I felt exposed — exposed for my ineptness, exposed in my nightgown.

All eyes were watching the dark monitor that suddenly jumped to life with a beeping green fluorescent line. First peaks of sinus tachycardia invaded the screen, a normal heart rhythm, but too fast. An occasional wide squiggle indicated that something worse was looming. The tongue-like waves of ventricular tachycardia marched across, then within minutes converted to the irregular hills of ventricular fibrillation -- not a good sign. Finally, flat line.

Gasp. Grunt. Chloe's body rattled the bed. The smell of a fart. Silence.

"Death has come," the doctor said and bowed his head. The medics collected their equipment and left. The doctor shook out the sheet and folded it smoothly under Chloe's chin. He said he'd send someone to collect her body. The door clicked shut behind him.

Silence.

I put down the wet washcloth and looked at my roommates who kept vigil around the bed. We looked as if we'd attended a pajama party and a prank had left us all tongue-tied.

Within ten minutes the door snapped open. A salt-and-pepper-haired woman entered the room and introduced herself as Phyllis, one of the facilitators for the workshop. She smelled of patchouli and orchestrated the bathing of Chloe's body, explaining that it was a ritual that Kubler-Ross encouraged to create closure for those present at a death, a way to show respect for the deceased. She talked about Chloe's death as no coincidence, but an example of *synchronicity,* when the inner and outer events in life coincided. "Your workshop has started early," she said matter-of-factly. "This week you'll figure out why you were in this room tonight." She handed out towels.

With Chloe's death my workshop began. I'd come to Arizona learn about dying, but also to have some time to myself. I did not expect to be called into action in the middle of the night before the workshop started. The burden of being a caretaker with all my current inadequacies was laid before me.

The workshop lasted for a week and included didactic information about the dying process and end-of-life care, as well as lectures from both Kubler-Ross and the physician who had attended Chloe's death. Some sessions were experiential, with opportunities to examine some of our own personal challenges, our "stuff," as they called it. Afternoons were dedicated to "mat work" where a small group worked with a therapist.

Phyllis facilitated my group. One woman banged out her anger at her absent father with a rubber mallet. Another sobbed into a pillow about the death of her child from leukemia. The rest of the group knelt or sat at the edge of the mat lending support. Sometimes it was simply witnessing "the worker's" pain; other times it was giving a hug or asking probing questions as the worker shared.

At the time this style of therapy was controversial, but Kubler-Ross believed patients often sorted through life's unfinished threads and traumas "the stuff" of their lives, during the dying process. By helping them understand the realities of their illness, and what could and could not be done to cure them, they were able to do a better job of planning how to use their final days. Working through the issues of their lives —examining old resentments and healing severed relationships made for a more peaceful death. The experiential part of the workshop, the mat work, focused on the living. Kubler-Ross emphasized that we did not need to wait until we were dying to deal with the thorns and resentments and disappointments we all carry with us. We should feel the urgency of living now, set our priorities, be honest about what is important, and move through our grudges, so that we can get on with living life fully in the present.

The mat work was hard for me. I was used to ignoring my feelings and soldiering on. My issues centered around self-esteem. I often felt inadequate. I could never do anything well enough or completely enough, and I was depleted. This was not my first emergency, my first ill patient, nor the first death I had witnessed, but somehow I felt responsible. As I shared these reflections with Phyllis during my time on the mat she asked me, "Why are you being so hard on yourself? You knew nothing about Chloe. You were not responsible for her." My expectations for myself were grandiose. I assumed I had much more control over patients and events than I did. I had unrealistic expectations for myself. In Arizona, I began to recognize my limitations; there was only so much I could and should do. I returned home to my work better able to move ahead in spite of my self doubts, to see my role as a facilitator, to realize there were aspects of healing and death I could control and those over which I had no control. I became a better listener.

***

Several months after the conference, I cared for Bill. A sixty-year-year-old gay man and a longtime smoker, he was dying of lung cancer. His wry sense of humor and gravelly laugh made him one of my favorites. After discharging him from the hospital, I kept in contact with him as a friend.

One wintry afternoon I visited him at home in St. Paul. A neighbor had shoveled the sidewalk to his bungalow, piling the foot of snow along the edge of the path. The chemotherapy was not benefiting him much, not slowing the cancer, just making him nauseous. He was deciding what to do. A rotund man, he filled the metal kitchen chair. As we sat at the Formica table, he told me about his conversation with his tumor.

"She's hot pink, very pretty. It's a she of course, but she smells." He chuckled. "I'm trying to build a wall around her, but she keeps jumping over."

"What is she telling you?" I asked.

"She says it's my time, time to quit fighting."

Bill enrolled in hospice, and I visited him at home on several other occasions. We chatted or sat quietly and I stroked the back of his thick dry hand when he was too tired to talk. He died within the month.

With Bill I began to understand the privilege I had as a doctor, to bear witness to life, the resourcefulness and the foolishness, the unexpected ways of coming to terms with the events over which we have no control.

***

Robert was a middle-aged mentally handicapped man brought to the hospital from the group home where he lived until he became critically ill. He was assigned to my team toward the end of my residency. Large, pale, and doughy, he had the acrid smell of illness. Blood tests and X-rays confirmed a diagnosis of sepsis — infection in his blood. We started him on antibiotics and admitted him to intensive care. After several weeks in the hospital he stopped eating and was losing weight. The infectious disease consultant posed the question: Should we insert a feeding tube so he could better fight the infection that racked his body?

With no close family, only an estranged sister, the state appointed a guardian to act as his power-of-attorney. The guardian, someone in a law office who had never met Robert, agreed to the feeding tube. But as his physician, I wondered if this was the right thing to do. Robert lay in his hospital bed, his eyes closed, uncommunicative. Antidepressants made no difference. The feeding tube would keep him from starving to death, but what kind of existence were we preserving? How much would he suffer? Could he even understand the pain for the gain?

I called his group home to get a sense of Robert. I'd only met him as a sick patient unable to communicate, and I wondered what was his life like before. I learned that he loved to sit at the table with his housemates and plunge into a plate of spaghetti. "Spaghetti's his favorite; he wears it after a meal." Then there was watching television with his house mates, especially Monday night football.

None of that was possible now. Staff would turn him every two hours in the nursing home. He had no visits from family or friends. It seemed more humane to allow him to die, without the tube. We'd keep him pain free, and nature could take its course. The guardian disagreed, so we took his case it to the hospital ethics committee.

I don't recall the outcome, but I do remember the fervor with which I made my point: this was not about curing. This was about death with dignity. Robert would suffer if we inserted the feeding tube, and it would most likely not save him anyway. As a healer I could not torture my patient.

***

Rita lay on freshly stretched sheets in her private nursing home room. The hum of her humidified oxygen was punctuated by the hiss of her continuous positive airway pressure (CPAP) machine, which pumped air through the tracheotomy tube in her neck. Her husband asked that a classical music station play during the day. Outside her window he had hung bird feeders, filling them weekly. Rita never opened her eyes and did not vocalize, but she was responsive to stimuli, like a pinch on the arm. The nurses turned her every two hours, bathed her daily, changed her diaper, fed her through a feeding tube, and suctioned her saliva. Her husband was convinced a cure still loomed, that some miraculous intervention would restore Rita to who she was before her stroke ten years earlier. He asked that we put her on vitamins, and he looked into treatment possibilities at the university. Every week on nursing home rounds he had a new request. The nurses reported these to me dutifully, but rolled their eyes.

Rita was a full code; her husband wanted her to go to the hospital, which was thirty minutes away, when her pneumonia did not respond to antibiotics administered through her feeding tube. "Give her that intravenous stuff," he said.

I mentioned my concern about her potential distress in strange surroundings if we moved her to the hospital.

But he was convinced she would recover, and he became angry if anyone questioned him. Silently, I cringed at the thought of performing CPR and pressing on her sallow chest.

It was ironic that with the assistance of technology, Rita outlived her husband. After his death, their children changed Rita's code status. She died in her sleep within the month.

***

I met Ethel twenty years after my experiences at the Kubler-Ross workshop. I had matured as a healer. She was well into her seventies, with a full head of gray hair, her skin wrinkled like an accordion above her plump frame. She smelled of lilac soap. As a result of the bone cancer she'd survived twenty years earlier, her left hip and leg were missing. She came to see me for abdominal pain one spring day; the lilacs outside were in bloom. After a CT scan, I diagnosed a tumor in her liver, probably cancer. We had a family conference in the office with two of her children to discuss how aggressive to be. "We can send you to a specialist to find out exactly what this is. That probably means doing a biopsy which would require some sedative," I told them.

She winced. "But do I need to know?" she asked holding her hand over the right side of her abdomen, the location of her liver.

"Mom, it might be nice to know," the daughter interjected.

"How would they do the biopsy?" the son asked.

I explained that the doctor would give her something to relax her, numb the skin over the area, insert a needle into her liver guided by the fluoroscope machine, take a little sample of the tissue, and send it to the lab to see what it was. There would be the risks of bleeding and infection. If it was cancer, then she could talk with the oncologist about treatment. That would mean chemotherapy, radiation, or surgery.

Ethel nodded and moved her hand from the right side to her left pelvis, where her leg had been removed two decades earlier. She slowly rubbed the area. "You know, I've been through this once before."

"We don't have to do anything," I reassured her, saying we could prescribe medicine to control her pain. We could consult hospice.

"Oh, I'm not ready for hospice," Ethel said. Over the years, Ethel had done some volunteer work for hospice so she understood what they offered. She said she needed some time to "put her ducks in order."

"Mom, are you sure you are okay with not knowing?" her daughter asked again.

Ethel set her jaw and said, "I don't need to know."

So I typed a prescription for pain medicine into the computer and invited Ethel to call me when she needed more. A month later, after she had arranged her will and the plans for her disabled daughter, we enrolled her in hospice. She died several weeks after that, surrounded by her family. Ethel had a clear mind; she knew what she wanted and how she wanted to wrap up her life. Her children respected her wishes and so did I.

***

We physicians must do a better job of helping patients die a good death and of modeling to our students how we switch from curing to facilitating a good death. There are important ways to assist patients and families at this point: managing pain, helping the patient and family understand that death is near, giving them choices about how they want to spend the final days. There are gifts that come at this time for all involved. Our Hippocratic Oath observes, "I will remember that there is art to medicine as well as science, and that warmth, sympathy and understanding may outweigh the surgeon's knife or the chemists's drug." Being asked to assist at life's critical junctures was why I had become a doctor. These glimpses into the universal human struggle and the concrete ways people deal with profound experiences rekindles my awe.

Wounded Healers

"Healing is in the wound itself."
--Anonymous

‡ ‡ ‡

Confessions

Primum non nocere. [First do no harm.]

I confess: I hurt people.

Mr. White lay perfectly still in his hospital bed except for his quivering left foot. I focused on the blue veins in his left forearm that wiggled back and forth like worms beneath his papery skin. The veins in his right arm looked no better. If I wasn't successful with his arms, I'd attack his ankle. With every jab the vein, slid away and Mr. White winced. When I finally pierced the rubbery surface, the vein exploded, making it useless, meaning I needed to try again. Three strikes and I was out ; then I'd ask someone else to try. I sighed in relief when my third attempt was successful in front of his elbow, but it meant he could not bend his arm. I apologized; Mr. White groaned and passed some gas. I left his room trailing apologies.

As a third-year medical student finally on the wards, I was not prepared for the pain I caused people. Through all the rigors of medical training -- the lectures, the hours with my cadaver, the evenings and weekends with my notes and textbooks, there was no discussion of inflicting pain. Pediatrics was the worst; making children cry, even scream was not what I had envisioned.

My skills would grow with time, but I agonized about patients like Mr. White who were victims of my target practice. And when did I quit trying? It seemed reasonable to ask for help after three attempts. I cringed when other students reported more persistence — "I finally got the IV started after six tries." There seemed to be some line, some appropriate number of attempts, some point between macho and consideration for the patient. How did I gain skill, manage my incompetence and respect the patient? Some days were easier; I became superstitious -- "Today is a good day; don't jinx it. Yesterday I couldn't get anything." Part of it was confidence — "I can do this; I will do this." The skill came with performing the procedure, perfecting the technique, which inevitably caused pain for my patients.

In the community hospitals, experienced nurses, "IV teams," started all the IVs. But in the county hospital, the medical students and residents did the deed. Sure, we had practiced on dummies and on each other, but that was different. The dummies didn't cringe or complain. With my colleagues, I'd taken my turn. For the rest of Mr. White's hospital stay, his bruised arms reminded me of my ineptness.

***

Sometimes the pain and discomfort I inflicted seemed more invasive. As a third year medical student in gynecology clinic, I struggled to find April's cervix to collect her Pap smear. "I'm sorry," I said. We had practiced on hired models and I had had no trouble on an earlier patient. But April's cervix eluded me, and the transition from the model, who gave me practical hints, to April with her laissez-faire demeanor was challenging. The attending physician let me struggle. Then April yelled and shimmied up the table. I recoiled -- maybe I should stop.

"We need your cooperation here," the attending said in a stern voice. "Scoot down to the bottom and put your hands under your buttocks." The attending grabbed April's hands and positioned them. "You need to learn how to do this," he said to me.

I repositioned myself on the stool. Tears filled April's eyes. I wasn't sure that I should continue, but I didn't want to cross the attending. I reminded myself to breathe and said, "I am going to touch you now." April said nothing. I reached toward her vulva, separated the skin, taking care that no pubic hair was caught, and slid the speculum into her vagina. Her cervix popped into view. I collected the specimens, thanked her, but felt uncertain about what I had done. Had we forced April to have the Pap smear?

The following week I confided in the therapist I was seeing.

"Why do you think you feel bad about this?" she asked.

I don't recall my response, but I struggled with the coercion; had we collected the Pap smear against April's will? Should we have quit? I'd held a child down to collect blood, but that seemed different. Gynecologic procedures and rectals were unpleasant. I remembered my first rectal, performed on an unconscious patient; the attending had directed four of us to do the procedure. All of us did as we were told, but felt bad afterwards.

What was the line between doing something for someone's own good and forcing them to have it done? How did permission work? I had gone to medical school, in part, to be a compassionate doctor. At the time, a fourth of my medical school class was female; women brought more compassion and personal experience to procedures such as Pap smears, the awkward position and all. I had expectations about what kind of doctor I would be.

"Look, you are human," the therapist told me. "Sometimes you hurt people, despite all your good intentions."

I wasn't sure she understood. She'd never performed a rectal or a pelvic exam, never passed a nasogastric tube. Was I okay with hurting people? Was there a way to hurt people with more compassion? This new role had many grays.

***

I confess: I hurt people in the process of healing them. Gradually I recalibrated my brain — sometimes pain came with the gain. I grew to realize that patients tolerated the hurting; patients had expectations given my role. But there was something about the manner in which I hurt patients, there was a way to ask permission and reevaluate it.

Primum non nocere -- first, do no harm -- a fundamental medical precept often assigned to Hippocrates (460-377 B.C.). However, this phrase actually departs from Hippocrates who said: *"to help the sick for the good of my patients according to my ability and my judgment, and never do harm to anyone."* Is that even possible? And even now, despite my abilities and judgments, patients don't always want what I have to offer.

***

During the last few years, I've cared for Debbie, a "difficult" patient with uncombed, mousey brown hair who squeezes her rolls of fat into her jeans. She usually "yes-buts" the suggestions I give her. Exercise — "I don't have time." Cut down on your soda pop — "It helps me function." Physical therapy for back pain — "it's too hard to get there." I've decided that she is depressed. Of course, she isn't interested in anti-depressants.

One morning Debbie came to see me with a new complaint. "I can't sit," she said. She stood, shifting her weight from one foot to the other. I had a medical student with me. Together we examined Debbie and identified a thrombosed hemorrhoid, a painful condition that could be remedied quickly. For once, I could help her.

We took Debbie to the minor procedure room, a large room with a gurney that moved up and down and a big operating-room-style light. After Debbie changed into a gown, I directed her to lie on her stomach. The student stood across from me, separating Debbie's buttocks to expose the hemorrhoid. I wiped the area with sterile solution. The sharp smell of antiseptic filled the room. I explained what I was doing as I injected the lidocaine. Debbie rested quietly as

I sliced into the hemorrhoid and popped out the clot, about the size of your little fingernail. We reviewed the follow-up care; Debbie thanked us and sauntered down the hall, one of the few times I'd seen her leave with a smile. Finally, I had helped her.

Several hours into the afternoon, Debbie called to say that the lump was back. Had I missed something? I relived the procedure. Had another hemorrhoid become thrombosed? I encouraged Debbie to soak in the bathtub. "If the pain continues, come back this afternoon."

Debbie returned at the end of the day as staff prepared to close up the clinic. Sure enough, another hemorrhoid had developed. Frustrated, I explained the situation to Debbie. She finished undressing as I mustered the energy and prepared the instruments for round two. The medical student tagged along, hoping to do more than watch. I filled the syringe with lidocaine and handed it to the student, directing him to slip the needle under the blue skin of the hemorrhoid. His hands quivered, but he did a fine job.

"That hurts," Debbie screeched and shifted on the gurney.

I apologized. "It's okay to make noise, but please hold still." I took a deep breath and directed the student to continue.

But Debbie had had enough. She rose up on her hands and knees like a horse bucking off its rider and screamed, "I won't let you do this to me again."

She was at least two times my weight, and the force of her response thrust us back. I felt as if she'd spit on us. The student dropped the syringe on the floor and hugged the wall of the room as he turned ghostly white. Debbie knelt on the gurney clutching the sheet around her bare bottom and sobbed. Her wails rattled everything in the room. Seconds felt like hours. What would the student think?

Approaching Debbie cautiously, I summoned my calmest voice. "This is your body. I won't do anything you don't want me to. But I'm worried that this will continue to bother you."

"No way," she bellowed in between tears. "I'm out of here."

She jumped to the floor; the reverberation from the impact rose like a wave in my exhausted body. She wasted no time in pulling on her pants. Then she grabbed her coat, hoisted her purse over her shoulder and stomped down the hall.

"Debbie, if this does not go away, you need to go to urgent care," I hollered after her.

"They'll have to put me under," she shrieked and continued her tromp toward the front door of the clinic.

Fear stricken, the student stared in my direction. I wanted to yell at the student, blame him for Debbie's response, but he'd done exactly what I told him. Her behavior wasn't his fault. Breathing to regain my own composure, I explained, "You didn't do anything wrong; don't blame yourself. You did a fine job."

The student stared at me, still pale. I knew without a doubt that this event would be the topic of conversation for the next week and probably for weeks to come. I could imagine the student sharing the fiasco with his cronies over beers, "Let me tell you about the patient who stomped out of clinic…" At least I'd not blamed him for her behavior. I could have been the nightmare teacher, a horrible physician. But I had censored myself.

The nurse entered the room and her eyebrows rose as she took in the disarray on the counter, the gown and sheets crumpled on the floor. "What happened?

"Debbie didn't want the procedure," I blurted.

"Obviously!" the nurse laughed. "She was pissed." The nurse began to clean up the room then turned to the student. "You'll never forget this one." Tossing the paper sheet and gown into the trash, she continued, "Dr. Zink's a good doctor, but it's not like on TV. Not everyone rides off into the sunset. Some days you're happy to just be done with your day."

Grateful for her wisdom, I thanked the nurse, picked the syringe up off the floor and threw it into the sharps container.

That evening I phoned my sister, also a doctor, still whirling from the emotion, confessing my concerns for the student, relieved that I'd held my tongue. We'd both had experiences where attendings had taken their frustrations out on the nurses or the students. Thankfully, I'd kept my ego out of it. "You were professional," my sister said.

Still I worried about Debbie until the student informed me that he'd seen her the following week when he was working with my partner. Debbie had brought in a sick child. "She walked and sat just fine," the student said. "I wondered if she even recognized me." Together we pulled up her medical record. There was no visit listed in the system for her since her outburst, and no visit to the urgent care.

Primum non nocer was crafted by physicians in the late 1800s, more than 2000 years after the death of Hippocrates. A phrase of hope, intention, and humility, it recognizes that human actions, even with the best intentions, have unwanted consequences. I bring my knowledge and experience. I bring hope and the intention to heal. I try to bring my best self to my patient encounters and to the students I train. Despite all this, I am far from perfect and I often wish that I had more control over the process and the outcome than I actually do.

End of the <u>Medical</u> <u>Deity</u>

There is no medical deity. During my generation of medical training in the 1980s the concept of a god-like, all-knowing physician was disintegrating. In 1999, the Institute of Medicine's watershed report *To Err is Human* dealt the fatal blow. It pointed out that preventable mistakes by medical personnel in hospitals killed over 44,000 patients a year, more than the number of annual deaths from suicide (34,600) and homicide (18,400).

Clinics and hospitals retooled and struggled to build a "safety culture." Medicine was turned on its ear. It became okay for staff to check and re-check each other's work. It was not only okay, but it was the co-worker's responsibility to ask questions if a physician's order did not seem right.

This culture shift should have been a huge relief to physicians. However, it caused us to recalibrate our thinking about apologies. And we had to learn another skill: how to explain to patients and families the collateral harm that can and sometimes does accompany our remedies.

During my residency, our care team studied Mr. Brown's chest X-ray. What looked like a snow storm obscured the bottom half of his left lung. The image of Mr. Brown lying on his left side showed that the white opacity had shifted and confirmed fluid in his lung cavity. We needed to insert a needle into his chest, draw out the fluid, and send a sample to the lab to diagnose the cause -- infection, cancer or heart failure.

By that time I had done a half-dozen taps. I explained the procedure and risks to Mr. Brown and his son — that causing a leak in his chest could necessitate inserting a chest tube. I helped them sign a consent that said that we had discussed the procedure, including the risks and benefits. As Mr. Brown sat upright, I painted his back near the lower part of his ribs with betadine soap, injected lidocaine to numb his skin, inserted a needle and sucked out two ounces of straw-colored fluid. Mr. Brown breathed easier. "All went well," I told Mr. Brown and his son.

Test results from his lung fluid suggested infection and I wrote the order for antibiotics.

Later that day, Mr. Brown was gasping for breath. Almost as pale as his bed sheet, he sat upright in his bed and sucked air through his open mouth. He had suffered one of the complications — his lung had collapsed. We explained the new procedure, obtained another signed consent and inserted a 1-centimeter diameter tube in his chest. It would remain there for several days.

Mr. Brown's condition worsened. He spiraled down-hill for reasons we could not figure out, and three days later, he died. Throughout Mr. Brown's decline, our team discussed the case with his son. We apologized for his father's death. Had the lung tap precipitated his decline and caused his death? Probably not. Still, I felt guilty.

Current research shows that it is best to apologize when something goes wrong. In the past, physicians made statements to downplay an errors in order to avoid a malpractice claims. This was driven in part by the medical deity mindset. Physicians decided what was best for the patient and presented the risks and benefits in a manner that recruited the patient and his/her family to the physician's way of thinking.

Now, physicians are encouraged to be transparent from the beginning: Be honest with patients when there is uncertainty about a diagnosis or treatment, when there is no clear answer about how to proceed. Provide as much education about the possible risks and unexpected outcomes of the different options. Be frank when one of the risks occurs or the course does not proceed as hoped. We are to say, "I am sorry. The treatment has not helped...This is what happened. This is what we are doing about it. We will keep you informed. Is there anything else you need?"

In this way, we can become partners with our patients and their families, taking into account their values and goals. We weigh the pros and cons of the many treatment options as best we can and decide how to move forward. Together, we negotiate the subtleties that separate illness from health. In an imperfect world, this is a good place to start.

Yet, how realistic is it? In the heat of a crisis, when a patient treads water in an ocean of fear or pain, the list of risks is long, and the probabilities are complex, how much can one hear and process? Patients and families hear what they want to hear. Sometimes, with non-English speaking patients, we have to talk through interpreters. These conversations can take time and are easier if a trusting relationship exists between the physician and patient. But establishing such a relationship is often impossible in today's disconnected health care delivery system, where a patient is admitted by an emergency physician and cared for by a hospitalist, neither of whom knows the patient. Patients, families and physicians yearn for black and white instead of the many shades of gray.

A wife tells me that she and her husband did not understand that heart bypass surgery might cause damage to the brain resulting in some dementia. Now, she watches over the retired engineer much like she did her children. She resents the medical team and is angry about the outcome.

An elderly woman tells me she is not using the cream I prescribed at an earlier visit. She had seen me for a vaginal itch. After an exam I prescribed estrogen. Thirty years of menopause had thinned her skin causing discomfort. When she came in for a follow-up I asked if the cream was helping.

"I'm not taking it. I read the entire package insert and it said I could get cancer."

I explained that was true, but at age 79 cancer was unlikely. "You won't be using that much and cancer is a long process. The increased comfort may be worth it."

Physicians are in an untenable position. It is impossible to cover every risk, to anticipate every possible outcome, to have perfect communication skills for the particular mindset of the patient and his or her family.

I confess, in reality, it is much easier to be the medical deity. Explaining the probability of a certain risk happening is a complex discussion, often too complex for some patients to understand and it takes time. As the medical deity, I am cloaked in authority and presumed control, I know what is good for the patient and that is what we will do. The patient will not question my wisdom or omniscience.

Playing the medical deity, however, does not work today. No physician can or should determine what is best for a patient. There are endless possibilities, and patients and families may have goals that are different from our own. Some may be motivated to eat right and exercise religiously; others may prefer to pay for a pill. Some are ready to die; others are willing to keep trying for a miracle. Given finite resources, we must help patients make the tough decisions realizing they involve messy conversations and negotiations. Perhaps that is where we start, one imperfect human to another in an imperfect world.

Reflections on an Untimely Death

Breathless from running to find me, her black eyes wide with panic, Lupita, the translator, blurted, "She's having a heart attack."

Immediately, I knew that Lupita was talking about Célia. I had checked on Célia twenty minutes earlier. She had been resting quietly in the in-patient ward of the small Nicaraguan hospital. The room smelled of ammonia as a woman mopped the lackluster ceramic tile floor of the dingy yellow room with scuff marks on the walls. Fluorescent tubes on the water-stained ceiling flickered and buzzed. Scattered around the room were cracked, white plastic chairs. Among them, six rusty bed frames sagged under plastic mattresses. Each held a patient surrounded by family, hovering like patrons at the stall selling corn-on-the-cob down the block. Families provided sheets and blankets, fed and nursed their loved one -- tasks the nurse was too busy to do, with supplies the hospital didn't have.

Célia's bed stood in the far corner under a grimy window. Her sister kept watch.

Earlier in the day we had done a hysterectomy for cervical cancer. The anesthesia had worn off, and she was restless, complaining of back pain. I asked the nurses to give her a pain shot. They sent Célia's sister to the pharmacy to buy diclofenac, a cousin of ibuprofen. When I checked Célia before my meeting, she had received the shot and was sleeping peacefully, her frizzy brown hair, fair by Nicaragua standards, uncoiled over her pillow.

As one of two doctors and several nurses who had volunteered for the medical team of this Minnesota nonprofit, I was here to screen for cervical cancer. We collected Pap smears, then carried the slides home in our luggage to be read by pathology technicians at the local university. Follow up and treatment of the abnormals were completed on future visits. The nonprofit sent a delegation to the community three to four times a year.

Nicaragua has national health care, but the wait to be seen is long and services are limited. Physicians are salaried to provide care in the government clinics, but most see patients privately as well, often the physician's home. However, the local gynecologist directs public patients to his private clinic, where he charges them for services that should be free. The local director of our organization, Luis, says, *"Este doctor es corrupto!"*

The nonprofit has worked with this rural Nicaraguan community for more than twelve years in health, education, and construction projects. As a member of the town for most of his life, Luis understands the needs of the community and guides the nonprofit in partnering with the locals; he knows their priorities. Prior to our arrival Luis hand-delivers appointment times. The dates that our brigade will be in town are announced on the radio. More than half of our patients walk several hours or bounce on a bus for the better part of a day to see us.

Of all our patients, Célia had the most troubling diagnosis. She came to her appointment Tuesday afternoon. Paul, the U.S. gynecologist, sat with her and explained the results of the colposcopy performed during an earlier visit. Lupita helped him explain why he needed to remove Célia's uterus. He drew pictures showing where the cancer cells were located and how they could spread unless surgery was performed.

"Este muy gravid," Lupita stressed.

Célia's sapphire blue eyes were serene as she heard this news. *"Tengo dos ninos. No quiero mas ninos,"* she explained in a soft voice.

At 35-years-old, Célia didn't want any more children. She asked a few questions and then agreed to schedule her surgery the following morning. I completed her history and physical and wrote admitting orders. She went home to gather a few things and settle her children, returning later that evening with her sister. The next morning the local nurses prepped her for surgery.

Paul removed Célia's uterus without a hitch.

Now Célia was three hours post-op. What was happening? I sprinted through the courtyard, down the drab hallway, remembering her smile when I'd checked on her in her hospital bed before surgery, and the reluctance in her step as I'd helped her climb on to the table in the operating room.

Célia's brown chest was bared; the local internist pressed his palms between her breasts performing cardiopulmonary resuscitation (CPR). The breasts that had fed her sons were exposed for all to see. Her wide blue eyes stared, lifeless. To my horror, no one was giving her mouth-to-mouth resuscitation. There was no emergency cart, no mask for mouth-to-mouth, no oral airway. A nonfunctional oxygen machine stood next to the bed.

Adrenaline coursed through my body, but my muscles froze. How to join in? I should give her mouth-to-mouth, put my lips to her lips, but I could not. My feet seemed glued to the floor. Other patients and their families gawked. How to create privacy? I didn't know enough Spanish to ask how to help or to ask for the tools I needed. Finally, in seconds that felt like hours, the local staff moved her into the operating room and the anesthesia technician put a breathing tube down her throat.

Now I could assist. With my stethoscope, I only heard breath sounds in the right side of her chest, so I directed the anesthesia tech to pull the breathing tube back from her right lung so that air could pass equally into both lungs. As I helped him tape the tube in place, a surgery nurse attached monitor leads to Célia's chest so we could check her heart rhythm. The monitor box showed a straight fluorescent yellow line. We checked that all the leads were attached. Still flat line. Another nurse wheeled over the defibrillator. The internist applied the pads to her chest and called, "*Claro*." Everyone stepped back from Célia. Her body jumped with the voltage.

No change -- flat line.

The local gynecologist arrived and slid into the effort. Over the years, Paul had tried referring cases to him, but he had not managed them appropriately, either repeating procedures in his private clinic so he could charge patients or telling them that our Pap smears were incorrect and reassuring patients that they did not need the treatment that we had recommended. Given this "corruption" we had quit sending patients to him and had worked with the hospital to identify gynecologists in another community. What were his intentions now?

I took over CPR, my palms pressed against Célia's warm sternum, trying to squeeze her heart: one and–press, two and — press, three and press . . . circulate the medications, stimulate her heart. It was a relief to see the Nicaraguan team follow the protocol familiar to me.

Wake up Célia I mumbled under my breath. One and two and three and . . . We worked together; not a well-oiled machine but we assisted each other.

At 4:45, Paul materialized, breathless and disturbed. I filled him in as I continued to push on Célia's chest. "Maybe a reaction to the med or a blood clot?" Paul fingered his collar. "Or bleeding from the surgery site?" He pulled on a latex glove and reached into her vagina, to check. The cloth sponges were barely moist with blood. His relief was palpable.

We ran the code for thirty minutes and pronounced Célia dead at 5:00 p.m.

The Nicaraguan team clustered together on the far side of the gurney and conferred in Spanish. Given our tenuous relationship with the gynecologist, we worried he could damage our reputation and make it impossible to continue our work here. Paul and I needed to know what the Nicaraguan team was saying. I grabbed Lupita by the elbow and traipsed over to the group. "Lupita, please translate," I urged. Paul followed us.

They were discussing internal bleeding. The local gynecologist wanted to check Célia's abdomen for blood. Someone handed him an 18-gauge spinal needle and 50-cc syringe. Authoritatively he bared Célia's abdomen and shoved the long needle in just above her pubic bone. If there was blood, it meant that Paul had missed a bleeding vessel.

Paul watched as if he was preparing to take an exam, sweat beaded on his forehead. He stared at the syringe, a slight twitch in his upper left eyelid.

The local gynecologist drew back on the plunger. No blood. A collective sigh.

I asked Lupita to help me tell the Nicaraguan doctors about the timing of the pain shot, given barely thirty minutes before Célia stopped breathing. Perhaps she had had an allergic reaction.

"But no hives," the local internist pointed out in Spanish after lifting the white sheet to examine Célia's body for red blotches.

"True, but sometimes hives are absent with allergic reactions," I replied.

"Perhaps a pulmonary embolism (blood clot in the lung)," Paul said. Célia's legs had been up in the stirrups for two hours. If we'd been in the U.S. we would have wrapped her legs with elastic bandages to prevent blood clots, but here there were no bandages to do so. In addition, Célia had been on oral contraceptives, which could have increased her risk.

The local physicians continued to converse.

Lupita motioned to me, then mouthed, "Célia's sister."

Paul and I trudged into the courtyard and collected our thoughts. During the day, the area was filled with staff. Now the area was quiet, empty, except for the janitor with his one glass eye, who pushed a pile of trash with his broom: dirt, crumpled papers and empty plastic bags with straws that had been containers for juice. Beyond the brick wall that marked the end of the courtyard, the trash smoldered. Whiffs of smoke floated by. After surgery, I had carried a clear plastic bag, filled with bloody gauze and paper drapes, and tossed it into the orange and gray embers. A few turkey vultures poking through the garbage at the edge of the cinders had fluttered in surprise.

As Paul explained the possible reasons for Célia's death, Célia's sister hung onto her friend, burying her face into her shoulder like a small child. She wailed and blurted words I couldn't understand between sobs, her thick body shuddering as if she had teeth-chattering chills.

I tightened my shoulders, pressed the hold button on the imaginary black phone and held my own emotions in check, "medical mode." There was no time to name the guilt, regret, sadness, even horror. I shoved away the myriad of feelings, and handed out tissues.

Célia's sister straightened her posture and pushed strands of dark hair from her face, She rattled on in Spanish, too fast for me to understand. Something about her mother.

"She doesn't know how to tell their mother about Célia's death. Their mother is ill. This will be hard for her." Lupita's voice trembled.

More rapid Spanish, more tears.

"They are also worried about a coffin. They are poor," Lupita said.

"How much does a coffin cost?" Paul asked.

"Two to four thousand *córdabas*," Lupita answered.

About $100-200 in U.S. dollars. Paul and I looked at each other and nodded. "Tell her we'll take care of this," Paul said.

We agreed to meet at the hospital later that evening with the money. The sister and friend hurried off to secure a coffin.

We returned to the operating room. The local team had decided that the death was caused by either an allergic reaction to the pain medication or a blood clot. Autopsies were not performed here. They reassured us, there would be no further investigation, but they'd call the medical director of the clinic. He'd want to talk with us. The local gynecologist helped Lupita and Paul write a note for the medical chart.

Within a half-hour, two men carried a tan metal coffin into the back hallway where Célia's body lay on a gurney draped with a sheet. Her Mickey Mouse-patterned quilt and her polyester dress and cotton panties and bra were folded at her feet. Paul and I pulled out the IV lines and breathing tube and removed the pads from her chest. Then we helped the nurses lift her naked body into the coffin lined with imitation white silk. I struggled to support the weight of her legs, her body odor already musty. A nurse double-checked Célia's wrist for a pulse, then covered her with the sheet. She directed me to tuck the faded quilt and clothes into the coffin at Célia's feet. The lid clicked shut.

A glass window sat in the upper part of the lid and was covered by a small door with a tiny knob. Lupita tugged open the little door and looked inside. I followed her to see what she saw. The window framed Célia's wide face and her halo of frizzy brown hair, her eyes now closed.

Two men lifted the coffin and carried it through the halls of the hospital. Adults and children sat and stood. Some were waiting their turn to be seen, others visited loved ones. Everyone's eyes followed the coffin out the front door.

The men set the coffin on a concrete bench just outside the building. Passers-by gathered, taking turns opening and closing the little door to peer in at Célia, as Lupita had done. Patrons from the corn-on-the-cob stand at the end of the block wandered down the street to look through the window in the coffin lid.

I stood near the front doorway of the hospital watching the parade. Were they showing respect? Or were they curious, checking to see who had died? Was anyone saying that this was the woman who the U.S. doctors had taken to surgery? No one glanced toward me; I was one of several standing near the front door. This was so different from my U.S. experience of death.

The stream of locals opening and closing the door in the coffin lid continued for about ten minutes. Then a large white pick-up truck with "Ministry of Health" painted on the door pulled around the corner and parked at the curb. Two men hoisted the coffin from the cement stoop, loaded it into the back of the truck, and hauled it away.

After the crowd had thinned out, Luis sat on his motorbike. His face was contorted as he chewed his cheek and played with the snap on his helmet. He'd heard rumors. After I summarized the events for him, he told me that he was worried about what this meant for our work. "I'll watch for reactions as I visit the communities," he told me. Then Paul rushed out of the hospital to find us. The clinic director had arrived and was waiting to talk with us.

Dr. Garcia, the clinic medical director, sat at his desk tipping his chair against a white-washed wall that held framed diplomas and awards. I had met him shortly after our arrival and was again struck by his youthfulness, mid thirties at the most. His stomach rolled over his belt, the sign of a higher income and a more sedentary life than most of the locals. Paul related the events as Dr. Garcia nodded and scribbled notes on a scrap of paper. Then he asked a few questions and Paul responded, reiterating concern about what this would mean for our work.

Dr. Garcia reassured that he'd talk with the family. "These things happen. *Esta bien.*"

***

I walked alone the five blocks to the restaurant for dinner. As I slowed my pace, my mind was flooded with thoughts. Why had I hesitated to put my lips to Célia's lips and breathe into her lungs? Was I afraid of catching something? My cheeks burned at the thought. Or was I afraid to insert myself too quickly into the code? The internist was in charge, this was not my world. If I had given her mouth-to-mouth, would it have made a difference? Would Célia have lived? In the U.S., a death so near a surgery would raise concerns about malpractice, but here no one brought it up. Had I been too demanding with Lupita? As our translator, she had stood in the middle of the crossfire? I had needed her desperately; my Spanish was inadequate; stress made me forget some of the vocabulary I knew -- Russian words popped in or my mind went blank.

Following a dinner rice, beans and chicken, Paul, Luis, and I returned to the hospital with the money for Célia's coffin. Célia's friend waited near the doorway of the inpatient ward, the site of Célia's code. There was no hint of the earlier drama; once again all six beds were occupied, each patient tended by family and friends.

We sought privacy again in the nearby courtyard. Paul expressed his sadness about the outcome of the surgery. Luis translated. *"Lo siento mucho . . ."*

Célia's friend described Célia as *allegre* . . . she filled the world with joy. "It was Célia's time. These things happen. *Sólo Dios sabe."*

Our absolution. Here it was accepted that some things ended badly, despite all good intentions.

Paul took a step back, perhaps still slogging through his guilt. Tears welled in my eyes; suddenly the dust from the street scratched the back of my throat. I prayed silently for the two motherless sons, the elderly mother now preceded to her grave by her daughter. Célia, her wide smile, frizzy hair, and sapphire blue eyes, only 35-years-old. Swallowing hard I struggled to control my tears.

Luis handed Célia's friend the envelope of money for the coffin. More condolences and good-byes, then our small group separated. Luis sped home on his motorbike.

Lost in our thoughts, Paul and I ambled back to the hotel, stepping in and out of the light cast on the dirt street from the open windows and doors. A soft rain dampened the ground and stilled the dust.

The Call Came

I remember the dimly lit room, the damp and musty smell of Mary's body, the rustling of the sheets and sighs as my patient labored to deliver her stillborn baby. In such situations, I can soften the loss with platitudes --"it wasn't meant to be," or "it's God's way of dealing with imperfections." But what can I really do or say in such a situation that doesn't diminish the powerful truth and honors the legitimate emotions?

I told Mary I was sorry and we cried together, but we still had to get through the drudgery of Mary's mounting contractions, her pain, my pain in watching her suffer.

I had followed Mary's pregnancy every month, listening for the heartbeat. We'd just begun measuring the growth of her uterus, one centimeter for every week. The curved edge of her uterus had become palpable above her pubic bone, like a growing cantaloupe. By twenty-five weeks it was well above her belly button. Then, I couldn't find the heartbeat. Was the equipment malfunctioning? I arranged for an ultrasound. Her baby was dead.

Mary was a teacher with a toddler at home and a supportive husband who painted houses. They weren't wealthy, but they desperately wanted to add another child to their family.

At the time, I was in my early thirties and completing my residency. I'd never been pregnant and did not have a significant other. I was on a career track — college, medical school, residency. I was in no hurry to have my own children.

"Don't you have a life?" Mary chuckled, then sucked water through a red straw.

"This is my life. I'm a resident. I'm on call," I said. "Besides, you're my patient."

Her humor made the unwelcome outcome easier for both of us.

***

And then there was Emily, one of my many pregnant teens whose mother had birthed her when she was about the same age as Emily. Each month Emily's belly grew rounder, well beyond Mary's cantaloupe, more like a watermelon. During the last month I saw her every week. First we chatted about how things were going, then I reviewed her vitals: blood pressure good, no protein in her urine, some edema at her ankles, her many rings a little tight. In the beginning, she'd hop up onto the exam table, but toward the end she lumbered. Emily always smiled when she heard the baby's heartbeat, the probe sitting to the right of her butterfly tattoo and the belly button ring with its fake diamond. At one point, I'd told her it was like "the rhythm of a galloping horse," and she reminded me of this at each visit. She called the baby "Pony."

"Please give her another name," I said as I wiped off the gel. She pulled her once baggy t-shirt down across her protruding belly and sat up. We reviewed elements of her preparations and plans: the necessity of a car seat, pros and cons of bottle or breast feeding, plans for contraception after the baby was born. I encouraged her to go to birthing classes, but she wouldn't. "My mom and sis'll be with me."

***

In modern times we have options related to child bearing: choose the timing of a child, let nature take its course, opt not to have children, assist the body in getting pregnant. Having children was not a given for me. I was the oldest of six; my two younger sibs had special needs, Down syndrome, so I'd already done my share of parenting. At age seven, when I knew my Mom was overwhelmed,

128

I rolled up my sleeves and pitched in. A "little mother," I learned to get points by helping her out and perfected my caretaking.

Only when I married in my mid-thirties did my childbearing desires kick in, mainly because my husband wanted a family. Then I realized I was terrified of having an abnormal child. My sister was married and pregnant as well. We were both terrified. What if . . . ? There was amniocentesis. There was abortion. After my Down syndrome sibs were born, my parents had the family genetics checked; we were not carriers of a chromosomal abnormality. Our fears were irrational, but very real. I had two miscarriages; my sister had two healthy children.

Others offered me the platitudes I'd shared with Mary. The miscarriages shattered the dream of family for my husband and me; the losses tore us apart instead of knitting us closer, and our marriage ended.

My parenting desires were still ticking, though, and I wasn't confident that my uterus could support a pregnancy without a lot of help. I didn't want to submit myself to being pumped with hormones and the invasive tests of modern fertility treatments. In fact, my family history and the irrational fear that my own uterus might produce a damaged child led me to think that adoption might be easier.

I identified an agency, paid the fees and completed the papers, asked friends to be references, and endured the home study. I had friends who had been adopted, but I knew no one who had been through the other side of the process, so I blazed my own trail, following the markers left by strangers. Somehow I survived the scrutiny: questions about my upbringing, my thoughts on parenting, discipline, finances and the home tour. Initially, I decided that I wanted an older child and turned to a friend who coordinated Russian adoptions. I fell in love with a six-year-old girl in a bleak Russian orphanage, but she was found to have something wrong with her and I suspected fetal alcohol syndrome. She was suddenly no longer available.

I decided that maybe it was better to look for a younger child. Vietnam had recently opened; a different agency, more paperwork. After a year, I was assigned a one-year-old boy, but the social worker described the red-tape the couple ahead of me had encountered -- several months in the country trying to get permission to bring the child home, appearances in front of authorities, possible bribes. Perhaps I was conflict avoidant, but I did not want to go through similar hassles, so I withdrew my application and pushed on.

I moved to a larger house that would have enough room for a live-in nanny. I wallpapered and painted the baby's bedroom in primary colors and bought a crib from friends of friends. I found a rocking chair at a local antique store. There had been one in my bedroom as a child, and even though I had no memories of being rocked, I'd watched my parents rock my younger siblings. And I'd rocked them too and sang silly songs.

The social worker presented pictures of toddlers in South and Central America -- Colombia and Guatemala, but those pursuits ended and I no longer remember why. I'd been on this adoption path for over two years. Patience had become my companion.

One of my patients told me about an agency in the U.S. which facilitated open adoptions of U.S. children; infants and toddlers were available, so I switched gears. My first "assignment" was an 18-month-old boy in Texas whose description was wonderful until I learned that his father, who was in prison, had not terminated parental rights. There was a chance that he would pursue custody when he was released.

Then one blustery Saturday morning in February, I flew from Minneapolis to Chicago, boarded the "L" to the Southside of Chicago with the address of the Gospel League house on a slip of paper in my pocket. I was on my way to meet Christine Nordenbrock. Her name sounded like it belonged to a tall and sturdy, blonde-haired German. In fact, she was a pregnant African-American in her early thirties, a recovering drug addict with three other children.

I climbed down the stairs from the elevated train station and trudged along the cracked city sidewalks. I zipped my down jacket, pulled my scarf up over my chin, and thrust my gloved hands deep into my pockets as I faced the bitter wind. The overnight bag, slung over my shoulder, slapped my hip with each step. Four- and five-story brick buildings with missing windows and doors were scattered between boarded up store fronts, a corner grocery store, a bar, and an auto repair lot filled with junkers.

Number 38 was a four-story building with peeling white paint. I pressed the buzzer to the right of the front door and announced my business to a metal box. A young, heavy-set woman greeted me expectantly, brought me into the foyer and paged Christine. Christine shuffled down the wooden stairs and greeted me with a broad smile that showed perfect white teeth. She wore a pastel turtleneck underneath a blue corduroy jumper.

I spent the rest of the day and the next morning listening to Christine's life story. The wind rattled the windows of her room that opened onto a view of the urban Chicago neighborhood where she'd grown up. The room's stark white walls held only a wooden cross which hung above the bed, no paintings or photos. Her Bible lay on the small bedside table. The worn carpet was cobblestone brown. She stretched out in an easy chair, her legs elevated on an ottoman, her jumper puffing out over her six-month pregnant belly.

Periodically she'd tell me "the baby's kicking" and she'd hold the corduroy taut so I could see her belly roll. She knew it was a boy.

Across the room in a straight back chair, I ran my hand over a white cotton bedspread; tiny knots marched across the bed in wavering lines. It reminded me of the one I had as a kid, the kind that when you fell asleep on it you awoke with stippled patterns on your cheek. Fingering the bedspread grounded me. A coldness gripped me despite my layers of long underwear, a turtle neck and a woolen sweater as I listened to Christine's story -- the different fathers, the drugs, the downward cycle. In her southern drawl, a legacy of the time she'd spent as a child with her grandmother in Mississippi, she told me, "My mother did drugs, I did drugs. It's in the family genes."

I thought of Emily whose "family genetics" seemed to predict teen pregnancy. Both Emily and Christine had made choices different from my own.

Christine's teenage son was now in juvenile detention, and her two daughters were currently in foster care. "Finally I hit bottom," she said. "You have to hit bottom." Alcohol, drugs, welfare and food stamps. Her life resembled that of many of my patients. She stopped using crack when she found out she was pregnant with this baby. "I found Jesus and got clean."

I shook off the chill. What did her actions mean for the health of this child, my child? According to the agency, all tests to date, including the ultrasound, showed no abnormalities. Given my upbringing childhood experiences, I was not choosing to have a special needs child.

After a lunch of turkey soup and cornbread, I met her daughters, brought for a visit by the social worker. They were well behaved and polite. One had her hair in cornrows that Christine had braided the prior week; the other had pig-tails decorated with a half dozen colorful barrettes.

That evening I joined Christine and her housemates at the service in the church across the street and heard the minister rally the congregation. "You can be saved. Take Jesus as your personal friend and savior." Folks raised their hands, palms skyward, then stood up and shared their stories. Christine told hers. I listened, my Catholic faith a much more private affair. Voices belting out gospel hymns vibrated through the folding chairs. A few folks paraded up to the front to declare that they would turn their lives over to Jesus. I prayed for grace and the courage to continue to walk this path toward motherhood. The service ended on a high note, the energy palpable, like the air before a summer storm.

That night I slept in a spare room, happy for the solitude. The next morning after breakfast, Christine and I talked about names and together we chose Gregory Nathan, a name I was fond of, and she liked; no family associations for either of us.

By the time I got back home, I was exhausted. Dreaming of Gregory, I put the final touches on the nursery, adding a blue dresser with white ceramic knobs, a colorful mobile of dancing jungle animals and crisp new crib sheets decorated with rainbows. I checked out books from the library with advice for a white mother raising a black child. I waited. I made plans. My mother, who lived in Ohio, would meet me in Chicago when I picked up my son. The staff at my clinic surprised me with a baby bag stuffed with diapers, pins, bibs, bottles, Wet-ones, most of the essentials.

The call came. I was in my office, a pleasant room even without windows. A Pablo Picasso print, the Blue Family, hung on the wall.

"Christine has changed her mind. She wants to keep her son," the social worker from the adoption agency said.

The piles of medical charts in front of me grew fuzzy as my tears welled up. I wasn't going to cry, not yet. I wanted to get off the phone as fast as I could. I thanked her for the information and dropped the phone in its cradle as if it scalded my hand.

***

"Focus and breathe. Breathe out the pain. Exhale now with the contraction. Slow. One, two, three . . ." Emily was a natural. I was relieved. Sometimes, without the classes, birthing becomes a horrendous screaming fest. But Emily pushed and strained with silent determination and concentration. Only once did she yelp in pain. The baby's bald head crowned, then emerged as I supported Emily's skin around the vagina so she would not tear. I suctioned fluid from the baby's nose. Miraculously, the tiny body rotated. I applied steady downward pressure on the head so the shoulder popped out, then upward so the other shoulder was freed. The baby slipped out, just as it was supposed to happen. I lay the baby on Emily's belly and toweled the white cheesy-like vernix off the pink skin, fisted hands and wiggling feet. A girl.

The cord needed to be cut. If a father were present, I would offer him the opportunity. Emily's mother was there, but busy admiring her new granddaughter. So I slipped on the clamps, sliced between them with scissors, applied gentle traction on the cord of the placenta and waited for its delivery. This family included four women: a thirty-something grandmother, who birthed her daughters as a teen, Emily's nineteen-year-old sister who had a three-year-old, and seventeen-year-old Emily whose newborn daughter's thin wail rose to greet an uncertain future.

***

I like to believe that Mary and her husband got pregnant again and added another healthy child to their family, but I lost track of them after residency. Emily and her sister were good mothers in their way, but they brought fewer resources to their parenting and needed society's support. Christine had even fewer assets; hopefully she continued on her new path of sobriety and was a good mother to Gregory Nathan. When I've looped through Chicago on I-94, I have wondered what became of her, of Gregory.

I, too, would have been a good mother, but after Christine changed her mind, I gave up. I could not ride the roller coaster of hope and disappointment again.

I can judge the choices Emily and Christine made in their lives, but what good does it do? Elevate me, denigrate them. At the end of the rant, I still held the hand I had been dealt.

I closed the door to the baby's room for a month, then one Saturday I wiped the dust off the animals of the mobile, wrapped them in tissue paper, and tucked them in a cardboard box. After removing the sheets and mattress pad, I folded them into a paper sack and disassembled the crib. I loaded the packages into the trunk of my Toyota along with the diaper bag full of baby items and slid the mattress and crib sideways into the back seat. I gave them to the local domestic violence shelter.

Back home I stood in the empty room and stared at the bare corner where the crib had stood. The absence of dust outlined where it had rested on the wooden floor. My voice echoed in the room as I cried and recited rote prayers that I had learned in Catholic grade school: *Hail Mary full of grace blessed is the fruit of thy womb . . . Holy Mary mother of God pray for us . . .*

Sometimes when I have no words and want something more than silence, this prayer fills my head. Since the call came, now more than a decade ago, I have found other ways of including children in my life: spending time with my niece and nephew, borrowing a friend's kids for the weekend, volunteering to parent a high-school exchange student from Korea, mentoring pre-med and medical students.

Not having the daily responsibility of parenting has opened other doors, but there is always an emptiness. What if . . . ?

On the Navajo Reservation

In an outpatient clinic in eastern Arizona, Navajos of all ages wait in a room without a television, so different from the waiting rooms at home where the television blares. Nurses shepherd patients into the exam rooms and I, along with the other physician and a nurse practitioner, try to address their worries and concerns -- a typical day. Outside the exam room window the sagebrush desert unfurls to orange and purple mesas that step up to oak and aspen covered mountains rising to greet the big sky. About a mile behind the clinic Canyon del Muerto cuts into the earth stretching several miles until it connects with Canyon de Chelley, a sacred place for the Navajo and a national park. I am here for several months, between jobs. In the east it rains, a ballooning black cloud is skirted by vertical gray streaks, but here the sun shines. We are at 8,000 feet; I am quickly winded when I run.

I pick up a chart from the plastic holder on the door; the complaint reads "weakness." Marge, one of the Navajo nurses, comes up behind me and says, "Mr. Anderson is one of the few authentic medicine men. The weakness is in his chest."

I knock and enter with Marge. Mr. Anderson is accompanied by two young Navajos, his grandson and his grandson's girlfriend. Their shiny black hair in identical pony-tails, tied at the napes of their necks, reaches to their waists. They are casually dressed in jeans and sweat shirts. In contrast, Mr. Anderson has dressed up to come to the clinic, as most elders do. A crisp denim blue shirt is buttoned at the neck with a bolo-tie clasped with a turquoise stone framed in silver filigree. He sits in the chair next to the desk, the skin of his face and neck the texture of weathered wood.

I introduce myself and extend my hand, palm touches palm, the Navajo hand shake. I mention the rain in the east and, perching on the stool in front of him, inquire about his weakness. Marge positions herself to my right, where I can watch her face, and she translates my question into Dinè (Navajo); her voice a low alto. She is middle-aged, her body thickened by five children. Now, a grandmother, she remembers boarding school days where, as a teenager, she was forced to kneel on the floor in her slip, the Caucasian priest pacing between the rows of young Native girls, admonishing them for speaking Dinè with each other.

Mr. Anderson responds in a soft bass. Navajo words seem to come from the middle of the tongue. I lean forward to hear the rhythm and imagine him chanting the healing hymns at ceremonies, a steady drone.

I ask his age.

"Somewhere past ninety, I think," Marge says.

No fevers, sweats or chills. His clothes fit the same. No chest pain, no shortness of breath. He eats all right. He's bothered by passing gas at ceremonies. His urine stream is strong. He performs ceremonies most evenings. His days are spent in prayer. When he sleeps, he sleeps soundly. He does not drink alcohol. He lives with his wife. There are six grown children.

Direct eye contact is uncommon among the Navajo and while we talk, Mr. Anderson looks at his lap. Traditional healers and medicine men intuit what is wrong and dispense with this oral history; I wonder if he is frustrated with me.

I suggest that it is time to examine him and ask his grandson and the girlfriend to wait outside in the waiting room. Mr. Anderson stands and shuffles his feet along the linoleum floor to the exam table; one hand holds open his eyelid the other grasps a carved wooden cane. He has the redundant eyelids of old age and in order to see he must lift his eyelid with his fingers. A little taller than I am, about 5 feet 5 inches with a "c" curve in the upper part of his spine, he hyper-extends his neck to look straight ahead. In his younger days he was probably as tall as his grandson, with the same long black hair. Now his hair is trimmed short and peppered with gray.

I examine him, following my ritual of palpating the scalp and neck, looking in eyes, ears and mouth, listening to heart and lungs, check his abdomen and groin. When I examine his genitals, I apologize. No edema in his ankles. No clues.

I ask more questions. As he speaks he sometimes gestures with his right hand. I imagine him in the hogan leading prayers.

"Do you have any worries?" I wonder how that translates in Navajo.

Mr. Anderson shakes his head.

I look at Marge, puzzled. "What am I missing? There has to be something. Could he be depressed? Would you ask him about finances, the health of his wife . . ."

Still no clues, I explain that we need to draw blood, to check his blood count and thyroid and then we will take an x-ray of his chest.

Marge guides him to these locations and I bring his grandson and the girlfriend back into the exam room in order to question them more. It is the girlfriend who tells me about the alcoholic son, an uncle to the grandson. This son banished Mr. Anderson and his wife from their heated home with indoor plumbing into their hogan this past winter. The hogan is the traditional home of the Navajo, a six sided building built with logs, the door opening to the east to greet the sun. People still live in them in the cooler canyon during the sweltering summers on the mesa. But now hogans on the mesa are generally reserved for ceremonies. I imagine this elderly couple trying to stay warm during the bitter winter, wind creeping through the cracks between the logs and mud. No electricity. No water or toilet facilities. I am suddenly aware that I am shivering.

When Mr. Anderson returns from lab and x-ray, I ask him about these problems with his son. Marge's face is stoic as she translates. "He steals stuff: money, baskets, blankets, jewelry, gifts and payments to Mr. Anderson for performing ceremonies. He sells them for alcohol. The son curses Mr. Anderson and his wife, yelling that his father's ceremonies are trash. The mother is a whore. They are afraid of this son." I watch Mr. Anderson's face, looking for a tear, some indication of his fear and frustration. There is nothing, he sits in the chair, periodically opening his eyelid to look at Marge as she speaks. The girlfriend leans against the white washed wall, wipes her eyes with a tissue; the grandson stretches his arm across her back, massaging her shoulder with his long fingers. Marge continues; her voice is low. "They're afraid he'll come home drunk and kill them. He has threatened."

Beneath the complaint of weakness, this.

I readjust my position on the stool. Outside, it is now raining; raindrops pelt the exam room window. What are the right words, what is the correct response, but I can only think to say, "I'm sorry that this has happened to you and your wife."

"There is no word for sorry in Navajo," Marge says.

No word for sorry; I'm not sure how to proceed; apologizing is how I was taught to empathize with a patient's pain. I blurt out, "Say what is culturally appropriate."

Marge utters something in Dinè.

While she speaks, I collect myself and find my professional demeanor. Girded again, I explain that abuse of the elderly is a mandatory report for me as a physician on the Navajo Reservation as it is in most states in the U.S. I must call protective services and I describe what this entails.

The grandson tells me that he and his girlfriend have moved back to the reservation and plan to stay with his grandparents who are now back in their house.

Relieved, I suggest starting Mr. Anderson on an anti-depressant. "It will change his brain chemicals and help his weakness." I delineate how to take it, possible side effects, and ask them to return in two weeks. "We'll see how things are." I offer my hand to each of them and we touch extended fingers and palms.

After they leave I walk to the nurses' desk and prepare to call Adult Protection. "Don't expect much," Marge says. Other nurses echo her concern. "You can call and report, but nothing ever happens." They explain that reservation officials are notorious for ignoring abuse, even in children. I pick up the phone and punch in the number which is posted on an important contact placard at the desk. The social worker who calls me back is familiar with the case. She tells me that their office has tried to file an order of protection, which means that the son could be arrested if he goes on the property. "But Mrs. Anderson has refused to sign it." There is nothing more they can do until the Andersons sign it.

I urge her to check out the situation again, pressing that Mr. Anderson is in frail health. "Maybe now due to her husband's health, Mrs. Anderson will sign."

"We can try," the worker says her voice flat and noncommittal.

I assume that the other sons have taken their turns, tried to intervene and failed. Now the grandson has returned to the reservation and is willing to confront his uncle.

In the evening I wait for the moonrise. The night before the moon was full. Beyond the clinic and its compound of ranch-style homes is a basketball court where the children of the clinic staff skateboard when there are no Navajo teens playing basketball. Walking past the court I am outside the range of the floodlights that light the clinic and compound drive. At the horizon line a luminescence sharpens the outline of the tabletop mesas on the right. Silently I stand and watch, listening to my breath. Inch by inch the sharp curved top of the moon appears. As it climbs, the shadows of the telephone and electric poles lengthen.

I pray for Mr. Anderson, holy man and healer, caller of the spirits. Afraid of his son, forced back into the cold hogan, the gifts from his ceremonies pilfered for alcohol and drugs, the toll his earthly troubles take on him.

I think of other wounded healers. My colleague in residency, who sniffed whiteout in the hospital bathrooms, deluded all of us until fatigue due to anemia interfered with her ability to care for patients -- her breaking point. She could no longer deny her addiction. Administrators forced her into substance abuse treatment.

My sister, a physician, married to an alcoholic for fifteen years denied his alcoholism, increased her drinking to pace his, until she learned of his two year affair. Only then did she initiate divorce proceedings.

I came to the reservation to heal myself. Exhausted, I needed a routine and the space to walk in the canyon, watch the sky, smell the sage, release the hold button on my black phone and process the swirl of feelings. Then I would start my University job.

Mr. Anderson, have I helped you today? With my black bag of remedies and healing, I prescribed medication, called protective services, and invited you back for a follow-up visit. I linked your fatigue to the course of events, listened to your pain. I cared. You and your wife are still faced with turning your son over to the police. Is there a breaking point at which you will take action?

There is my own blindness and denial, a lifetime of wounds still sore despite my on-going efforts to seek a full 360-degree self-knowledge.

A light breeze and the sagebrush suddenly perfumes the air. Now a slightly lopsided moon balances in the sky. As healers we may try to escape our humanity, think we have a special status, but we are not above being human, cannot escape vulnerability.

The Gesture

For some time, I had been interested in working for Doctors Without Borders (DWB), an international organization delivering emergency medical aid to those in need. On the day that I finally arrived in their New York office a young nurse grilled me with pointed questions about my coping abilities. It was the most grueling interview ever and this was a volunteer effort!

Several months later, I was invited to a week-long orientation. From dawn to midnight, along with several dozen volunteers, I was introduced to DWB's mission and procedures. Since I had done some consulting in Russia I was invited to consider Chechnya. The head of the Chechnya mission happened to be in New York at the time testifying at the UN about Russia's war crimes in Chechnya. A meeting was arranged at his brother's apartment.

I took the subway to the neighborhood and found the rent-controlled building. As I climbed the stairs to the fourth floor, I wiped my sweaty palms on my black jeans. Jeffrey greeted me at the door. Tall and thin he had an aquiline nose and wire-rim glasses. He charmed me with photos of Chechen and Ingush staff on his lap top. There was instant rapport.

The computer hummed as one photo faded into another with the push of a button. Jeffrey gazed at the computer screen and smiled. "Rules are we go nowhere unaccompanied." He glanced at me. "These are our guards. I eat dinner with them every night. I've gotten to know them quite well." His long finger pointed. "Adam, Nazir, Mugamed."

Three olive-skinned faces grinned at me. One was blonde with a mouthful of gold teeth. A second had coal-black hair; I guessed they were in their late twenties. The third was older, a receding hairline with gray at the temples.

"We've done a lot of rehab work," he said "and with your help we can improve the care given to patients."

"The trauma hospital is in Grozny, the capital of Chechnya. This is the surgical suite, or theater, as they call it. Before . . ." The skeleton of a cement-block room filled with rubble and blown-out window frames appeared. "And after." In the next photo, the debris morphed into shiny white-tiled walls and sun poured through glass windows onto a surgical gurney and steel instrument table.

Jeffrey explained that Chechnya had been mired in war for centuries. For the last decade, Chechens were fighting for independence from Russia. It was a simplification of the facts, but Russia wanted to hold on to Chechnya because an oil pipeline coursed through the middle of the country. Grozny and a number of other cities and villages were destroyed during the mid 1990s.

"Doing something gives them purpose," he elaborated. "We build trust, then we can implement new practices. While DWB delivers supplies and monitors their distribution, we count injuries from land mines and guns and collect stories of the ongoing human rights abuses."

"Such as?" I asked.

"Such as locals trying to get medical care, who are delayed at Russian checkpoints. One was a pregnant woman in labor. And young men who are fighting age are arrested for no reason." Putin had declared the war over, but it was not. There were daily acts of terrorism, car bombs, and abductions. He handed me a security brief. "Read this," he said, "then we'll talk."

On the plane home I reviewed the document. Five years ago, six international aid workers were murdered in their beds in a Grozny hospital. That stopped all aid operations in Chechnya for a year. Since then, five years of security breaches: muggings, robberies, kidnappings. Despite these, Jeffrey had restarted efforts over the last year.

Within the week we talked by phone and Jeffrey patiently answered all my questions. Friends and family questioned my sanity — "A war zone?" At forty-five, single and childless, I was ready to take some risks to do some good. I trusted Jeffrey. I signed the contract for Chechnya. I would leave in a month.

During that month, I ran my first marathon, moved my belongings into storage, finalized my will, settled my dog with my parents, and flew to Amsterdam. For three days I met with DWB managers who oversaw the mission. I went to Moscow for a few days, where I met with DWB support staff and set up a home base in one of the DWB flats. Then Jeffrey and I flew to the airport just outside of Nazran, Ingushetia, about thirty minutes from the Chechen border. Nazran, the capital of Ingushetia, was a safer province and was our base for operations in Chechnya.

We lugged our baggage down the rickety stairs to the tarmac. After walking fifty feet, we stepped through a tall wire mesh fence and into a crush of people. I struggled to stay close to Jeffrey. Nazran staff found us quickly and led us to two white cars with DWB logos. Jeffrey greeted the men, brushing cheek to cheek and introduced me. Staff shook my hand.

We would ride with Nazir, one of the guards. Dressed in army greens, his rifle slung over his shoulder, he reminded me that this was a high risk mission. Smiling broadly, he took my back pack and helped me into the backseat with Jeffrey. After stowing our gear in the trunk, Nazir jumped in front next to the driver. Body scents were pungent. As we sped and bumped through the countryside to Nazran, Jeffrey pointed out refugee camps. One claimed space in six abandoned train cars, another in an old brick warehouse, and the third a shantytown of corrugated metal.

We drove through downtown Nazran. The center was marked by a roundabout framed with a mosque, two or three-story brick city buildings, and a dozen stores. In a neighborhood, the driver braked abruptly in front of an 8-foot metal gate with decorative filigree. He honked and the gate slid open, disappearing behind a brick wall. We pulled onto a thirty-foot patch of black top that separated two 2-story orange brick houses. They belonged to the town baker and his family who lived in the right-hand building. Our living quarters and office were in the house on the left. To reach the second floor everyone climbed stairs past my bedroom windows on the first floor.

I was relieved to have my own bedroom, the old kitchen. I stowed my few belongings in the broom closet and relished my private sink. My bed was a couch covered with a matching plaid duvet and pillow cover. On a plain formica kitchen table, I set photos, my journal, and Russian grammar texts. There were three other rooms, bedrooms shared by other aid workers, and a living room with a television and couches -- the center of our evening activities. The only bathroom could be reached through this room.

We ate most of our meals in a cluster of cement block rooms off the back of the baker's house. There was a picnic table covered by a plastic red checkered cloth. A dozen wooden stools were aligned around the edges. Adjoining was a storage room that was converted into a gym.

Long days usually meant we ate dinner at nine. I joined Jeffrey in his evening routine with the guards. Weary of meat and potatoes, I usually had tea and bread with cheese that squeaked in my teeth.

The men ribbed me about my bird-like habits. Conversations centered on the guards' stories about their lives and their animated inquisitions about us. Approaching middle age, with no spouse or children, we were curiosities.

One memorable evening Adam told us how he "stole" his wife. With a mouthful of gold teeth, Adam sputtered on in Russian, spraying bits of potato on me as he looked me in the eye.

"Stole?" I asked, horrified.

"Bride stealing is common." Jeffrey laughed and translated the tale. When it was time to enlist in the army at nineteen, Adam and his brother crafted a plan: His brother would pick up Adam's sixteen-year-old sweetheart when she was walking home from the market and bring her to him. He waited in the field at the end of their road. When she arrived, he kissed her and shot off his Kalashnikov, sealing the deal.

I stared in amazement. The candle glow shimmered in Jeffrey's glasses as he explained that by stealing a wife, Adam had avoided marriage negotiations and payments to the bride's father. "They wanted to get married. Sometimes the girl doesn't even know the guy."

Mugamed was a neighbor who worked part-time as our guard. Occasionally he brought his grandchildren to see me for medical concerns, a rash, or breathing problems. When he had evening duty, he joined us for dinner. He usually sat around the corner from me pulling out my stool and pouring my tea. Jeffrey refused to translate some of the things he said to me. "You don't want to know," Jeffrey said, raising his eyebrows.

A month into my mission, Jeffrey was abducted. He was on his way into Chechnya to deliver money to rebuild the obstetrical ward of a Grozny hospital. Overnight the medical supply mission morphed into crisis management. We did not know if Jeffrey was dead or alive. Aid deliveries ceased in Chechnya; finding Jeffrey became our focus. Now I was living what I had read in the eleven-page security brief.

A European DWB management team swooped in to assess the situation and control the crisis, completely underestimating the importance of our relationships with our Chechen and Ingush staff, especially the guards. Kidnapping 101 was not a course in medical school, but I knew it was imperative to keep an ongoing connection with the guards. Having dinner with them and conversing through a translator did not recreate the intimacy we had shared when Jeffrey was there. I was dependent on a translator for anything beyond the pleasantries.

One day a solution presented itself. Exercise was imperative for my sanity and running outdoors was not an option in Nazran due to security. Knowing my exercise addiction, Jeffrey had encouraged me to purchase an exercise bike in Moscow and ship it to Nazran on a supply truck. I put it in the storage room off the kitchen where aid workers had rigged a pseudo-gym. The eclectic room had many functions, containing a weight machine from a predecessor, a refrigerator for immunizations, a Muslim prayer rug used by the cook and some of the guards, and a potbellied stove for warmth. Daily I pedaled out my frustrations, either in the early morning or before dinner. I often studied my Russian while biking. One morning Nazir wandered in and gestured at my vocabulary text.

He grinned broadly, read the verb and conjugations and encouraged me to repeat them after him. He enunciated syllables that I struggled with. After a while, he grew bored with the verb tenses and began teaching me the names of objects in the room.

Pointing to the ceiling Nazir said, "*Potolok.*"

I repeated, "*Potolok.*"

Then he pointed to the floor, "*Pol.*"

I said, "*Pol.*"

This continued until we had identified most of the items within the room: door, corner, prayer rug, refrigerator, chair, boxes, even the barbell with its pipes and disks.

From then on whenever Nazir or Adam was on duty, I had a tutor. They were task masters, quizzing me on what we had gone over the time before. The camaraderie was important, especially since Jeffrey was kidnapped.

Nazir usually smoked a cigarette while he helped me. Being a non-smoker, this annoyed me and I thought about asking him not to smoke. Many aid workers and staff smoked. Smoking was permitted on the porch and stairs to the office. Entering or exiting the office necessitated holding my breath through the fog. Jeffrey had asthma, so no one smoked in our office or house. But since his kidnapping, DWB managers were more lenient about allowing smoking in the living room.

With no progress in securing Jeffrey's release, the DWB managers decided that it was too dangerous to have an American in the field. Without warning I was ordered to return to Moscow. I had twenty-four hours notice to say my good-byes. I was leaving staff in the lurch. Furious, I felt like a plant ripped from the earth, vulnerable roots exposed.

That evening I paced the black top inside the compound trying to make sense of their precipitous decision and come to some peace. On duty, Mugamed paced with me, but sensing my despair and need for silence, he respected my distance, only murmuring as he fingered his prayer beads. The air was chilly and I reached deep inside the pockets of my parka for some morsel of wisdom. I gazed at the inky black sky sprinkled with stars asking for grace.

Yanked from the field, my hopes to do some good were now impossible. Was this program a waste of time? Health care in

Chechnya was no better. The local staff continued to struggle with daily threats to their friends and family. What had I accomplished?

Step. Step. The snap of my shoes sounded against the pavement, answered by the echoing clicks of Mugamed. My breathing slowed and deepened. Somewhere between those sounds, I found a place for my heart to rest. Somewhere between my breaths, I realized that it was my intention that counted. They would remember the effort, the human connection, the shared laughter. They would know that an American had helped, that I had made a gesture.

Postscript: Jeffrey was returned unharmed twenty-six days after his abduction. Over the next two months, the program was phased out and disbanded due to security. DWB has slowly restarted efforts there. Listed as one of the ten most underreported stories by the media during 2005, many Chechens have not returned to their homes. Russian officials claim the situation in Chechnya has normalized. Much of the capital, Grozny has been rebuilt. Modern office buildings and apartments replace the skeletal remains from the wars. But car bombs, detainment at checkpoints, kidnappings and murders still occur.

Circle Back Home

Hal, a wiry man in his mid sixties who sometimes took the time to shave, shook his head and set his jaw. "So I have to have a stroke before they do anything?"

My impatience simmered. We'd gone through the facts several times. Hal did not have enough blockage in the artery in his neck to make the surgery worth the risk. "The most important thing you can do is quit smoking and take your daily aspirin."

"Hrumph! Can't do that." Hal rubbed his nicotine stained fingers together. His son who sat next to him smiled; it was the first time I'd met one of his kids. Hal didn't want to have another stroke. He'd had the surgery on his right carotid artery several years earlier. Now he wanted to have it on his left.

Hal and I had been through a lot in our three year relationship. The first year I convinced him to admit his alcoholic wife, disabled by a stroke, to a nursing home. "She's wearing you out. You can't do this anymore. You have your own health problems." Always a "hrumph" from Hal. He wore his exhaustion like a rumpled shirt. Too much cooking and cleaning, and sometimes she didn't make it to the bathroom in time. When she was in the nursing home and no longer his responsibility, he couldn't shake his guilt and battled depression. Hal pushed my patience to its limits with his *hrumphs.* Now I was evaluating him for dizziness.

***

Several days later, after another visit spent reassuring Hal, the phone startled me awake. My clock flashed 6 a.m. I wasn't on call. Who needed me? Wind rustled the window panes of my bedroom as I fumbled in the darkness for the phone. It was Eileen, my sister's partner, calling from the Caribbean; they'd flown there Christmas day. No *hello, how are you*, just: "Amy had a stroke. She can't walk. We're at the hospital in St. Lucia."

I sat bolt upright. Not Amy! I was the oldest of five girls. Fifty-year-old Amy was eighteen months younger than I. We'd struggled with sibling rivalry well past adolescence. Her bigger-than-life-personality had been a challenge for me. I struggled to find the lamp and almost knocked it over as I switched it on. "What happened?"

Eileen pressed on. "We had a great first day of vacation. The island is gorgeous. Last night Amy got up to go to the bathroom and fell out of bed. She couldn't walk. I woke up the owner of the bed and breakfast." Eileen's voice cracked. A successful businesswoman, who worked in finance and traveled around the U.S., Eileen, with her calm logic, was a perfect yin to my sister's yang. Eileen swallowed tears as she described the drive up the hill to the old hotel that housed the hospital. The emergency physician had examined Amy and ordered a CAT scan. "Now we're in a hospital room. The admitting physician just stopped by. Will you talk with him?"

Vibrant and active Amy, who usually skipped, was now unable to move her arm and leg! If she had been in the U.S. she would have received the clot-buster drugs that often limited the deficits from stroke. She had no risk factors. She didn't smoke, didn't have high blood pressure or elevated cholesterol and wasn't on birth control pills.

Forty-eight hours later and $45,000 poorer because Amy had not purchased medical evacuation insurance, she was admitted to the service of the premier stroke neurologist at the University Hospital in Ohio. After a variety of tests, we learned that she had a dissection of her right internal carotid, a major artery off the aorta that carries blood to the brain. The lining of the artery tore had torn, causing blood cells to stick together along the tear and form a clot. A piece of clot had broken off and travelled to the part of her brain that manages the sensation in the left side of her body. With the blood supply blocked, the brain tissue in that area was deprived of oxygen and no longer functioned. The damage could not be repaired.

***

I saw Amy and Eileen before they noticed me. Amy slumped slightly to the left in her bed. She was not using her left arm or leg. No make-up, no pierced earrings; her complexion was sallow; she exhibited all of her fifty years. Her blonde hair was pulled back in a ponytail. She dressed in a t-shirt and gym shorts, no bra, too hard to fasten. Eileen wiped Amy's mouth with a tissue. This was so different from her groomed and coiffed professorial self, lipstick and an unusual pin on her suit jacket lapel as she stood at the front of her college classroom.

I forced a smile and stepped into her room. The fragrance of the spring bouquets on the windowsill blanketed any smell of illness. She smiled when she saw me; tears welled in her chocolate brown eyes. I was glad I'd made the trip from Minnesota to support her. Little did I know how important my advocacy would be and what insight I'd gain into my profession.

As always, Eileen was neatly put together, but her weariness manifested itself in the creases around her hazel-green eyes. Together Amy and Eileen updated me: Amy was waiting to be discharged to rehab tomorrow. Her mood was subdued and she worried about how Mom and Dad were dealing with the stroke, how our sister with Down syndrome was coping, what her recovery would entail. I steeled myself against the onslaught — I'd come to help.

After some small talk, we settled in for the evening. I opened my maroon roller-bag in the corner of the room and dug out my red plaid flannel nightgown. In the glow from the streetlights, seven floors below us, I spread out the hospital sheets and cotton blankets on the couch and stuffed the hard pillow in its case. As I crawled under the covers, one of the lilies in a bouquet released a whiff of fragrance.

I breathed deeply to calm my racing mind. When I was a child and teen, Amy 's embellishments got me in trouble. I'd told her that I tried marijuana in college. She informed my parents I was smoking daily. She raved to acquaintances about something I'd accomplished, and I found myself making excuses and backpedaling. "It's not quite that way . . ." In gatherings she held court, played the jester, and topped others' anecdotes. I was exhausted when I spent much time with her. Here I was face-to-face with one of the most difficult members of my family. I didn't really trust her. Somehow competition for the approval of my parents had persisted into our fifth decades. We were too old for this. Now she was wounded. I fell into a sleep of fitful dreams.

The following morning Amy, Eileen and I sat in the room with our Starbucks coffee. With the morning news shows chattering in the background, we prepared for the medical team's morning rounds. Amy had the beginning of a headache. She followed in the footsteps of my mother who had had trouble with headaches as long as I could remember, especially when stressed. Before the stroke, Amy took an aspirin and caffeine combination up to five times a day. Since this was no longer an option with her blood thinner, the medical team was struggling to manage them.

The neurology resident entered the room and greeted us. He looked like a college freshman, too young to be at this stage in his training. He asked how things were. Amy described the headache.

"Can you start her on a low dose tricyclic at night to prevent her headaches?" I apologized for butting in, explained that I was a family physician, spelled out the similarities between Amy's and our mother's headaches, and our mother's relief with these medications.

"That's an outpatient issue," the resident replied curtly.

Miffed, I let the headache issue pass since we were planning on discharge later that day. He completed a thorough neurologic examination. I swallowed hard as I saw her flaccid left arm and leg and the excess bounce when he checked her reflexes; she could talk, her mind seemed fine, but her physical mobility losses were huge.

The day slipped by with therapy appointments for Amy. The hospital social worker assured us that all was in order, but when 4 p.m. came and went, we realized that we weren't going anywhere. Again, Amy felt a headache starting and asked for medications which she received. I knew she'd fall asleep, so I left and drove the hour to visit my parents. At 9 p.m. Eileen called to tell me that the social worker from the rehab hospital had finally called. "She said it's an insurance problem," Eileen explained. "The University hospital never processed Amy's insurance, so the insurance company doesn't know Amy is here and can't approve the transfer." Eileen sighed.

I settled my parents the best I could and drove back to the hospital early in the morning so I'd be in Amy's room when the physicians made their rounds. The young neurology resident was on schedule, and I explained the insurance issue. "Not our problem. Talk with the social worker," he told me and repeated Amy's neuro exam.

Taking a step toward the bed, I persisted, explaining what the hospital social worker told us yesterday and that I'd left her a message when we discovered the glitch. "It's almost nine and we haven't heard from her."

The resident shrugged. "She's probably in a meeting."

Amy asked for pain medicine for her headache.

"I'll have the nurse bring you some Tylenol," the resident said and slithered out the door, off to his next patient.

Amy burst into tears. Eileen stepped to the bedside to comfort her. I told Amy and Eileen that I'd talk with the attending physician when he checked in. A few minutes later, a middle-aged orderly arrived to take Amy to physical therapy. Amy mopped her tears with a handful of tissues and then handed them to Eileen. She smoothed her hair with her good hand and asked me to help her slip on her terry cloth bathrobe. The pain melted from her face as she turned on her charm and addressed the orderly, asking him about his family and how long he'd worked at the hospital.

Eileen rolled her eyes as Amy left the room. "She's amazing, the energy she gets from people."

I agreed and encouraged Eileen to take some time for herself. Afraid we'd still be sitting in the room the next day if we didn't do something, I called the patient representative.

One hour later, I sat alone in the room working on my laptop when the neurology attending stopped by. "I know family members who are doctors are a real pain," I apologized. I explained the headache issue, asked about a tricyclic. He agreed with my plan. Then, I described our discharge problem.

"I'll put some pressure where I can," he said cordially and left the room.

Shortly after that, the social worker arrived and talked through gritted teeth. Obviously the patient representative had called her. She stopped short of an apology, but said all the right things and explained that she wasn't aware of the insurance issue.

I'd been in her shoes, so I tried my best to be kind despite my exasperation. I emphasized, "We need to move today. The medical team is done with us. They've more or less washed their hands." The social worker nodded and backed out of the room.

Late that afternoon we were on our way to the rehab hospital. We gave half of Amy's floral bouquets to the staff members who had been especially kind to her. Eileen and I lugged the other six bouquets down the long hallway and into the elevator, through the spinning doors and into the car, a 2-mile drive to the rehab hospital, unload, and then up a floor and down another long corridor into Amy's new room on the rehab wing of another hospital. Amy had charmed every staff member we encountered on our way to her room: the orderly pushing her wheelchair, the volunteer at the information desk, the director of rehab, and then her nurse. Eileen rolled her eyes at me as Amy worked her magic with the cleaning lady who checked the towel supply in the bathroom.

The next day Amy was oriented to rehab with appointments all morning. Eileen took the morning to settle things at home — bring Amy "normal" clothes, feed their cats, check on the mail. She looked drained when she returned. "The voicemail's full. I couldn't deal with it," she told me and began to unpack Amy's clothing.

Amy continued in what I've called her "extreme extrovert" mode, asking personal information of every therapist, cleanup person or transport aide she encountered. She always found some detail to relate to: someone they knew in common, some advice she could give regarding the child ready to go to college. Eileen had asked the rehab doctor to limit visitors and incoming calls, but we had no control over how Amy interacted with staff. I'd lived with this since childhood, and when she was like this, I wanted to turn her volume down. Slide the dial to off, shut her up.

Now four nights away from home, two of those on the pull-out couch in Amy's hospital room, one evening calming our agitated parents, and the last night tucked into the recliner in Amy's new room, I happily anticipated leaving the next day. For dinner the three of us shared carryout from a local Chinese restaurant and then prepared for bed. As I covered my recliner with a sheet, the odor of cashew chicken lingered and we talked about the low-key atmosphere here in rehab.

"It feels more like . . ." then Amy's words slurred.

I spun around and stepped to her bed, grasping the metal guardrail. Amy's smile grew crooked. She could not complete her sentence. Eileen bolted to the bedside; her hazel-green eyes now brimmed with panic.

Tears pooled in the back of my throat; I choked and swallowed. My heart hammered in my ears; my feet were lead against the cold linoleum, my palms moist. I found my breath, sucked it in deep to summon my composure, and located my physician self. "Amy, smile for us."

She could not. Her eyes reminded me of a cornered animal frozen in the beam of a searchlight. She tried to talk, choked on her words and started to cry. Eileen dabbed Amy's eyes with the edge of her own t-shirt.

If Amy lost her ability to speak . . . I rushed into the hall, grabbed her nurse and explained what was happening. The rehab doctor stood at the counter charting. They sprinted into the room, examined Amy and ordered a CAT scan. A major concern was the blood thinner Amy was taking to prevent the extension of her stroke. If her blood was too thin, she could bleed into another part of her brain.

Seconds stretched to minutes. Amy's slurred speech and the crookedness of her smile disappeared. "I am so scared," she said clearly.

A wave of relief coursed through me -- thank God she could talk again. Did I ever think I'd wish that? While we waited for staff to take her down to radiology to have her CAT scan, Amy confided: "There are some things I need you to know. If this is it . . . I don't want to be a vegetable . . . " Her voice quivered, "Let me die."

Eileen paced, pausing to touch Amy's forehead, adjust a loose strand of hair.

"Ask Fathers George and Rick to say my funeral mass."

Automatically, I grabbed a legal pad from my backpack, dragged a chair close to the side of her bed, and pressed my pen to the page of yellow paper making notes. Songs, prayers, pallbearers, all the funeral details and how to care for our disabled sister. It took an hour to get it all down. When the orderly finally arrived to wheel Amy off for the head scan, I was numb.

Eileen and I sat in the sudden stillness of the room; the sound of Amy's gurney grew distant. Voices echoed from the nurses' station. "What's going on?" Eileen asked.

Tears hung in my throat again. "I wish I knew," I managed to say. "The worst scenario is that she's bleeding into her head, the part of her brain that controls her speech. But if so, her speech would not have come back. The scan will give us an answer." I leveled my voice, but my heart raced like I'd main-lined a cup of espresso.

Within the hour, Amy returned. "I'm getting used to this," she said as the orderly and nurse helped her slide from the cart back into her bed.

Eileen moved to her bedside and pulled the sheet and blanket to Amy's neck, tucking them around her limp left arm and shoulder.

Amy continued with the funeral talk, now focusing on her fellow faculty and students who would each need a personal call. "There's Stacey. Eileen, you've heard me talk about her. Sheeee . . ." Her words slurred.

I bolted from my recliner and clutched the cold metal guardrail, my palms sweaty. Her crooked smile was back, her eyes frantic. I thought of her first roller coaster ride. Maybe six years old, Amy's eyes were wild with terror as the car hesitated then fell down the first hill. She clutched the bar and screamed. Now her eyes remained frozen with horror, her face flattened on the left. She could not speak. How bad could this get?

Eileen, usually composed, touched Amy's cheek; her hand trembled, and she began to cry. I swallowed splinters and fumbled for the call button, found it, pushed it -- hard. When no one came, I dashed out the door to find the nurse.

As the nurse trailed me back into the room, the episode subsided. The nurse called the on-call doctor. While we waited, the end-of-life talk resumed. "I can't imagine living as a vegetable," Amy repeated. "Don't let them do that to me." I pictured Amy with a plastic tube in her throat, unable to talk, a machine pushing air into her lungs; I could not imagine it either.

The on-call doctor came in; he was professional and kind. "I'll check on the CAT scan. Her blood is anti-coagulated in an appropriate range. I'm not sure what's going on, but I'll ask the neurologist to see her in the morning. Until then I'm moving her to a step-down bed where the nurses can monitor her more closely."

We disassembled the room that we'd arranged a mere twenty-four hours earlier. Another trip down an array of hallways and elevators and finally at 1 a.m. Eileen and I were stretched out in new recliners to the beep of the telemetry machine. Amy was already asleep. Too exhausted to sleep, I tried to meditate on the invading rhythmic bleeps and found myself caught between restless sleep and nightmare dreams: I was on-call at the hospital, there were too many patients, multiple medical emergencies were happening simultaneously, I couldn't find what I needed, couldn't get anyone to help me. Finally, as gray light peeked through the slats in the shades, I struggled to pull on my running clothes and headed down the hall for a jog with the hope of clearing my mind.

The hospital doors twirled behind me. My Sauconys slapped the damp sidewalk silvered by the drizzle of a January rain. I saw Amy's crooked smile, her words slurring. Panic in her eyes; my palms wet against the cold metal rail. This sister whom I'd wanted to throttle, whom I've yelled at: "What did you tell Mom and Dad?" "You said what?" "Oh please, how could you?" All of this was gone, behind me. Slap, slap, slap.

When I returned, Amy and Eileen were awake, but tired. Amy's speech was normal. We discussed my parents' visit later that morning and decided it was best to delay it. I called my parents and explained Amy's speech episodes, the uncertainty of her condition and suggested they come later in the day.

Outside, the rain continued, a steady drizzle. Amy slept as Eileen and I sat in her room and worked on our computers. Mid-morning, the on-call physician stopped by and reviewed Amy's status: her blood was thin, but not too thin. The CAT scan was negative. Amy had had no more episodes, a good sign. The neurologist would come by sometime today. I was scheduled to fly home in the afternoon, but I was anxious to meet him and hear his assessment of the evening's events before I left. I'd cared for stroke victims but had never seen these kinds of events occur.

At noon, I asked the nurse if she'd heard from the neurologist, assuming he would have rounded early. She offered to page him. We waited. At 1 p.m., the nurse checked on us. She still had not heard from the neurologist, so I asked her to call again. I tried to be patient; I'd been there, trying to balance patient care and family obligations when on call. We waited and hoped. Sitting on the other side, facing the uncertainty, the not knowing, experiencing the vulnerability, subjected to the brokenness in the health care system, a system where I earned my livelihood and trained future practitioners. As a physician, I had advocated for Amy, but what about families who had no one who was medically trained.

At 2 p.m. the nurse reached the neurologist. "He won't be in today. He's coming tomorrow morning." The nurse frowned and shook her head.

This neurology team had been highly recommended. "But he was consulted last night at midnight."

The nurse nodded in agreement, her lips pursed. I knew this look and usually felt great empathy for the nurse caught in the middle, making excuses for the physician, but this was my sister.

"Will you call him and ask him if he'd at least talk with me before I fly out?"

She called and informed me that he refused to talk with me. "He wants to examine the patient before talking with family." Expressing her remorse, she echoed my frustration and anger.

It was beyond time to leave for the airport. I said a tearful good-bye to Amy and Eileen. We hugged, holding tight a few seconds longer, then I grabbed my roller bag and rushed down the steps to the front of the hospital. I hailed the first taxi I saw and pressed an extra $10 into the driver's hand for shuttling me to the airport in time.

***

Amy never had another episode. Although the first weeks were filled with worry, life settled into a new routine. She didn't regain the use of her left side. After three weeks in rehab, she was discharged to home with therapy several times a week. Over the next weeks, she learned to walk again and practiced an array of exercises — finding beads buried in clay, zipping zippers and fastening buttons--to recover the fine motor movement in her left hand. I talked with her, frequently making suggestions about how to work with her array of doctors: the physiatrist who supervised her rehabilitation, the neurologist who managed her stroke, and a psychiatrist she'd seen for years.

"Amy, choose one doctor, the one you trust to manage your headaches." She grew frustrated with her physicians who did not have the answers she desperately wanted. "When will the sensation come back? Will it come back?" She had trouble tucking in her shirt on her left side and could not put the backs on her pierced earrings. As someone who prided herself on her appearance, these disabilities were hard to take.

When her physicians met with her, they didn't talk to Amy but to the person accompanying her. "So I've got a disability and they think I've lost my mind! Can't understand," she complained. The physiatrist was late for appointments, confused her with another patient, and forgot that Amy had only lost her speech transiently. When Amy met with the neurologist, he had not yet reviewed her MRA, the study that showed the blood flow to her brain. She desperately wanted the blocked vessel to open, "so my brains get juice from more than one place." Despite being a stroke expert, he could not outline the roadmap to Amy's recovery. Most stroke research was on the frontal lobe of the brain, and he didn't know as much about the less common strokes in the parietal lobe which Amy had suffered.

I tried to reassure her. I understood the physician's uncertainty and confusion; I'd been there — too many patients, trying to keep everybody straight. I tried to explain this, but at the same time, I heard Amy's distress and hoped that I was not as impolite and inattentive with my patients as her doctors appeared to be with her.

Eventually Amy found a primary care physician who helped her coordinate the information from the specialists and manage her headaches. Amy searched Medline and the Internet, found a researcher who was working with parietal lobe deficits, called her on the phone and purchased her manual. She took the manual with her to therapy; the therapist copied it, cover to cover. Amy's neurologist asked her how he could get a copy. She found six articles that evaluated the benefit of electrical stimulation for recovering fine motor skills. I suggested she write a paragraph summarizing the studies and give it to her physician to incorporate in the letter asking insurance to cover the necessary equipment.

Six months later, Amy was back to work. She had figured out how to partner with her physicians. She understood that they were limited in what they could tell her; the research hadn't been done. They didn't have the time to do the literature review that she had done, so she educated them.

"Think of this as a new body, very different from the one you inhabited the first fifty years of your life," I told her. "It'll take some time to get to know it." I realized this image worked for her when I heard her repeat the analogy to me again and again.

***

A few weeks after Amy's stroke, I stood at the guardrail of Hal's hospital bed and watched him struggle to swallow his saliva and organize his words. Now the vascular surgeons would slice open his carotid artery, the big artery connecting his heart to his brain and, like a roto-rooter, clean out the blockage; Hal would finally get the surgery he wanted. Should I have pushed for him to have it earlier, though the evidence did not support it then? Did Hal have some intuition? Did I miss something?

Several weeks later in the clinic, Hal had his surgery, recovered and worked with speech therapy. His speech returned to normal, but he was sad and depressed. "I can't sleep," he complained. I checked blood tests, put Hal on anti-depressants, and asked him to return to see me in a week.

At the next visit I asked how he was doing.

"Hrumph," he shook his head. By all parameters Hal had been fixed or cured, the probable cause of his transient stroke symptoms now removed. I tried to convince him to stop smoking, but that was only one of my worries; he continued to lose weight. The road to recovery was long. I second guessed myself and rearranged his anti-depressants. He felt a little better and started to do his woodworking, then sliced off the tip of the index finger on his right and dominant hand. We were back to the beginning—his weight dropped, he was not sleeping. Such suffering. What would heal Hal?

Scientific evidence tells us how to manage stroke and treat depression, but little science guides my response to Hal's broken heart. How do I address the grief and guilt related to his wife's placement in the nursing home, his torment related to his own health?

Both my sister and Hal wanted direction about how to heal, assistance from their physicians with their struggles to become whole again. As I clutched the cold metal guardrail of Amy's bed, Hal's bed, I became a better sister, a better doctor and a better human being. What Amy's physicians did not give her at critical times was compassion, one human being to another. Although I had no pat answers for Hal, I did not flinch while he shared his despair. This in itself was probably as important as the medicines I prescribed or the consultants I referred him to. Human being to human being I listened to his troubles.

Faced with suffering, the pain and miseries that afflict a human life, I can sit, listen, and acknowledge the inadequacy of the tools in my black bag. It is the sitting with him, being present physically and emotionally, that will bring — not the cure, but the healing.

I remembered my sister in her hospital room. "It's scary," I told Hall. "You don't have a road map. This is a new body. You've not done this before." Hal did not have Amy's intelligence or curiosity about his deficits or his healing, but he still wrestled with the acceptance of what he could not control.

Gradually both came to terms with their losses. Healing came for both Hal and Amy. As I struggled to be present for each of them, to recognize their great effort as they plodded along their weary roads of recovery, I discovered that the healing went both ways. What was uncontrollable in my own life lost importance, and a new acceptance of life's challenges and my sister's and Hal's foibles washed over me.

Epilogue

I tugged open the heavy wooden 'Women Only' door of the Moscow *banya* (sauna), housed in a majestic, old building in downtown Moscow near Tverskaya, the shopping street. The men's entrance was around the corner. A cathedral ceiling with stained glass windows crowned the foyer. During the day, a mosaic of colors danced across the marble floor and up the marble staircase that twisted to the second floor where the larger of the two saunas was located.

Moscow was headquarters for the Doctors Without Borders (DWB) mission in Chechnya and Ingushetia, located two hours south of Moscow by air. I had an extended weekend break in Moscow after several weeks in the field. Exhausted from being "on" twenty-four hours a day and fed up with the erratic water and electricity at our Ingush compound, I was desperate for copious hot water and several hours of relaxation. I checked my coat at the wooden kiosk where a gray cat lay curled in the far corner, quietly licking herself. Some self-nurturing, just what I needed.

My weary legs tackled the marble stairs, forty steps to the second floor, then through shuttered doors into the restaurant thick with cigarette smoke. I held my breath through the fog until the glass doors leading to the *banya* slid behind me. Only then I exhaled with a deep sigh. A middle-aged woman with henna-colored hair and cherry-red lipstick refused to crack a smile despite my Russian pleasantries. She was "old school," making no effort at friendly customer service. Piling a towel, sheet, felt hat, and slippers on the counter, she pushed them toward me and then collected my wallet, watch and earrings to secure in a locker behind her. In my kindergarten Russian, I asked for a "wet massage." With a dour expression, she scribbled what I assumed was my name on one of three clip boards and directed me to a numbered spot on a long wooden bench in the changing area across the room.

Reminded of how limited personal space was in Russia, I undressed and organized my three-foot bench space. I tucked my boots under the bench, draped my top and trousers on the metal hanger above, hung my coat on the hook, and set my bag with shampoo, lotion and hair brush on the bench. I donned my flip-flops, wrapped myself in a white sheet and followed a tiled hallway into a gymnasium-size space.

Stained glass windows positioned in the upper half of the two-story tiled walls filtered the sunlight, creating patches of red, blue, yellow and green on the walls and cement floor. An ornamental metal gutter carrying water from the variety of showers and tubs ran along the base of the wall toward decorative drains. The area smelled of soap; the air temperature felt pleasant on my skin. Several elevated pools of cold water reached by ladders were scattered about. Showers were clustered off to one side. In another corner stood the wooden sauna that stretched two stories. The strident voice of the sauna mama shooed a procession of sheeted women out the sauna door into the larger room so she could perform her scheduled hosing down of the cedar walls and benches.

Throughout the room, carved stone benches supported clusters of women. Some bent over colorful plastic basins applying facial masks. Others were stretched out, shaving their legs or grooming their feet. Some women were alone; others bunched in small groups, deep in conversation. A circle of women sat off to one side holding books. Titters of laughter echoed throughout.

In the far corner, separated by a white linen curtain, was the wet massage area. The masseuse, a portly woman, wore an open, white, terrycloth robe over her white underpants and bra. Her green flip-flops slapped the black plastic mat under her stone massage table. I handed her my loofa (natural sponge); the colleague who introduced me to the *banya* had urged me to bring my own.

Massages had become an essential part of my *banya* ritual, and this time I'd chosen the wet massage. Three options were available: The traditional Swedish massage in a private room, where the masseuse kneads the body with oil. The birch twig massage occurs on a bench in the upper deck of the wooden sauna. Here the masseuse swats the naked and reclining recipient with small twigs and leaves pulled from a bucket of eucalyptus oil, while others in the sauna watch. This sauna is not on my personal list, but it is a popular choice. And finally, the wet massage; this was my second time.

In Russian and with gestures, the masseuse directed me to lie face down on the table covered with a red plastic mat. I turned my head to watch her preparations. She removed her robe and wrapped a white towel around her thick waist. First testing the water temperature with her foot, she sprayed me with warm water from a green garden hose. The droplets tickled. Soaping my back, she rubbed the muscles of my neck, then worked my shoulders. The soap smelled like my grandmother's lye-ash recipe, which I had helped her make when I was a child. I associated the fragrance with laundry, washboards, cleanness and sheets dried on clotheslines in the sun.

The masseuse scrubbed me with the loofa, scouring every inch of my back. I became a small child in the bathtub being bathed by my mother. Then I was dirty from play on my grandmother's farm; now I was burdened with the suffering of patients and colleagues in

Chechnya. Rubbing the muscles of my arms, elbows and wrists, the masseuse pressed her calloused fingers into my palms, working the small muscles and bones. She pulled my fingers, snapping my knuckles. Prickly vibrations spewed from my hands releasing the tension in my neck.

My mind wandered. . . I tried to remember how long it had been since I was really touched? Months, maybe years? No intimate relationship for a while; good men were hard to find. Relationships seemed to elude me. I interspersed international work with employment in the states. Without a spouse or children, I had the flexibility to take a leave of absence to do this mission in Chechnya. I'd always wanted to work overseas for an extended period of time, and this was the longest I'd ever been away from my obligations at home.

Raised in an upper middle class home and the oldest of six children, two with special needs, I learned how to work and care take from a young age. That germinated into becoming a doctor, which utilized and further developed my caring, listening, and problem-solving skills. There was a satisfaction that came from helping others. Sometimes it was safer to take care of another than to ask for what I needed and to risk rejection.

Now the masseuse massaged my shoulder muscles again, where my stress was rooted. As she pressed near my shoulder blades, I exhaled, pushing my stomach against the mat and table. I visualized the knot of tension in my trapezius and rhomboid muscles loosening. With my inhale, I directed breath between the muscle fibers.

Shortly after high school, in a yoga class, I'd learned the power of my breath. Since then, I ground myself by breathing and consciously pulling myself into the present moment. I visualize air filling my lungs then flowing into my torso, legs and feet and I bury it at least a yard into the surface beneath my feet. I do this frequently throughout my day -- when I talk with a patient, when I need to focus in the middle of chaos, before a presentation--I breathe deep and ground.

"Holodni?" the loofa masseuse asked. Not waiting for my response, she rinsed my back again and covered my buttocks with a towel. She elbowed the muscles in my back along my spine. The pressure smarted, but also felt good. She removed the towel slid her elbow into the muscles of my buttocks and along the edge of my gluteus causing intense pressure bordering on discomfort. I breathed and it released. There is a narrow margin between satisfaction and sting. Much of my life involves tiptoeing along that tight rope.

All life's pleasures: food, alcohol, sex, work, even play can become burdens that shift into vices. Dating the guy who was the life of the party had been rollicking fun, but marrying him? His ego had held an edge that gradually sliced at my own self-esteem. After two miscarriages, that marriage ended in divorce. Then came the messiness and pain that were the soil for growth. Freedom from that marriage had allowed me to accept and create opportunities to build my work life and travel, to decide to volunteer on the DWB mission. But there was a loneliness that came with being single, unattached . . . a deep loneliness.

Now the masseuse kneaded my thighs, rolling the large muscles with the palms of her hands. She switched to the loofa, scrubbing my legs; her force bordered on roughness. On this mission I had been surrounded by people twenty-four hours a day; the loneliness was nonexistent. I carried the stories that my Chechen colleagues shared with me. I absorbed them like a cloth absorbs stains; they could not be scrubbed out or wrung out. Loved ones killed during the war -- mothers, fathers, siblings. Families faced with daily threats of terrorism — car bombs, buried landmines, roving checkpoints where they were detained for no reason. These challenges were so different from those I faced in the U.S. Did my own problems and pain count? In comparison, my worries seemed miniscule.

The masseuse tapped my shoulder and motioned for me to roll over. I searched for the strength to lift up on my elbow and used the momentum to catapult myself onto my back. Shafts of light poured through tiny windows in the vaulted ceiling. My slack body sank into the mat and my contracted muscles no longer caused me to hover an inch above it. Current worries and challenges had ebbed away. Beyond the curtain I heard women's voices. Someone was singing. In the distance the sauna mama summoned the *jenchina* (women) back to the sauna. Her cadence resembled a call to prayers. I realized that the new age music which often played during massages at home was absent, and I had not missed it.

With another spray from the garden hose, shudders erupted throughout my body. Waves of relaxation broke like waves lapping the ocean shore, water running backwards and sucked into the sand. The masseuse soaped and scrubbed my front -- working chest and breasts. I lay naked, completely exposed, and yet felt enveloped in an aura of soap suds and healing.

Her thick fingers deftly localized a sore spot in my foot; the pressure edged on pain. Pressure. Hurt. Breathe. Focus. Breathe. Release. With the attention of the masseuse's fingers, the burdens of seeing and hearing suffering, carrying miseries, unraveled and released. As she focused on a knot in my calf, another wave of relaxation rippled through me and the tightness softened. A rinse with the hose and warm water spilled over and off my tingling skin and troubled psyche.

The masseuse mumbled in Russian and I realized she was finished. I lay there for a moment trying to find my legs. I stumbled off the table struggling to steady myself. Feet planted on the mat on the floor, I reached for my sheet. How to thank her? *"Spaceba,"* I bowed. *"Bolshoi spaceba."* I did not have the words to say more. This was a holy place, a temple to celebrate the body, to heal the heart and nourish the spirit. For now, my head was clear, my body relaxed, my thirst quenched, and my chasm filled. To heal and care for others, it was imperative that I also care for myself.

References

Shining Light in Dark Places

Child abuse facts accessed from http://www.cdc.gov/ncipc/pub-res/CMFactsheet.pdf

The Pilgrim's Journey

Kiecolt-Glaser, JK, McGuire, L, Robles, TF, Glaser, R. Psychoneuroimmunology and psychosomatic medicine: Back to the future. Psychosomatic Medicine Journal of Biobehavioral Medicine. 2002;64:15-28.

National Institute of Mental Health. Depression Can Break Your Heart. 2002. http://www.medicinenet.com/script/main/art.asp?articlekey=21761. Accessed March 3, 2012.

Nordenberg, T. The Healing Power of Placebos. FDA Consumer magazine January-February 2000. http://findarticles.com/p/articles/mi_m1370/is_1_34/ai_59111154/pg_2/. Accessed March 3 2012.

Whooley, MA. Depression and cardiovascular disease: Healing the broken hearted. JAMA.2006;295 (24): 2874-81.

Discussion Questions

<u>Overall</u>

Does the metaphor of a primary care clinician as a sin eater work for you? Why or why not?
Reflect on the changes in health care delivery over the past decade or two. How have they affected you or your family?

<u>Bearing Witness</u>

1) How does poverty affect one's health?
2) How might poverty result in health disparities?
3) As a health professional, what supports are in place in your community or practice setting to help you manage patients who are poor?
4) As a health professional, what supports are in place in your community or practice setting to help you manage patients who are narcotic dependent?
5) As health professionals, what can we do to create an environment for honesty with our patients?
6) Do you have an honest relationship with your provider? What works or what does not work about the relationship?
7) As a health professional, what are your responsibilities related to reporting suspected child abuse or child neglect in your state? Which other professionals have similar responsibilities?
8) Why might child abuse have an intergenerational component? (example, children who are abused as children and/or witness the abuse of their siblings or a parent and then grow up to repeat the pattern)
9) As a health professional, what is the value of spending time in health care settings in other cultures and/or in other countries?
10) What health care practices in the U.S. might seem odd or unusual in other countries?

11) When practicing in another culture, how do you respect the culture and yet practice "good" medicine?

12) Why were Dr. Musa (Second Opinion) and Dr. Miguel (Reborn in Honduras) important to Dr. Zink? What role did they play? Have you encountered individuals who have played the same role for you in other settings?

Mystery

1)   What mysteries or miracles have you experienced in your own life or in your work with patients?

2)   Have you encountered unexplainable events in your life? How have you interpreted them?

3)   What role does faith play in your life? What role does faith play in the life of some of your patients?

4)   Has anyone close to you lived with abuse in his/her intimate relationship? What did you learn about abusive relationships?

5)   Have you had a close relationship with an animal? What has that relationship meant to you? Why are pets used for therapy or as visitors in nursing homes or group homes?

6)   Discuss the possibilities of why Daniel's mother lost custody of him (Meeting Daniel). Have you had experience with or do you know children or adults who have been involved with the child or adult protection system? If so, reflect on the benefits and challenges of that safety net.

7)   What role has denial played in your own life? How was it protective? How was it a barrier?

8)   What role has addiction played in your own life? What role has addiction played in the life of someone close to you?

9)   Consider the death of someone close to you. What was that experience like for you?

10) What is synchronicity? Describe a synchronistic event that occurred in your life or the life of someone close to you.

11) If you are in a health care profession, recall the death of one of you patients. What was it like for you?

12) What is the value of an advanced directive? Do you have one? Why or why not? What works or does not work about an advanced directive?

13) In order to carry out the Hippocratic Oath: "Apply all measures that are required, but avoid the twin traps of overtreatment and therapeutic nihilism," physicians must be honest with patients about the choices they have. However, honesty does not guarantee an easy death. How can a physician or health professional help family, friends and/or patients with the dying process?

14) Some patients and families are in denial about death and choose to initiate treatment to cure when there is little hope of such. Others simply need honest information about what is possible along with the permission to call it quits. What are your experiences with these realities?

15) What rituals of death have you experienced in other countries, and/or other cultures? What did you learn from them?

Wounded Healer

1)   As a health professional, how have you come to terms with the fact that sometimes you cause pain when you are trying to help patients? Is this expected due to your role? Reflect on the statement: "But there was something about the manner in which I hurt patients, there was a way to ask permission and reevaluate it."

2)   As a patient, when has a clinician hurt you in a manner that was acceptable? In a manner that was unacceptable? Reflect on the difference and why?

3)   As a health professional, reflect on your experiences with giving informed consent. What are the challenges and how do you manage them? As a patient or a family member reflect on receiving or hearing informed consent. What was it like? What was clear or unclear about the procedure and its risks and benefits?

4)   As a health professional, has the care you've given a patient resulted in a bad outcome? Reflect on what you learned from the experience.

5)   As a patient or the friend or family member of a patient, have you experienced a bad health outcome? How did the clinicians and those involved deal with it?

6)   Describe a loss in your own life. What did you learn from it? How did you heal your heart?

7)   What lessons did you learn when you spent time in a culture different from your own?

8)   As a health professional, how have interactions with your family informed the care you provide to patients?

Acknowledgements

The Gesture won the 2007 Pilgrimage Writing Award and was published in *Pilgrimage*, Colorado, 2008, Vol 32.

A shorter version of Living and Dying Well was published in the *Anthology Twelve Breaths a Minute*, Southern Methodist Press, 2011 and then re-published in *At the End of Life: True Stories of How We Die*, Creative Nonfiction Books, 2012

The following stories were published in *Minnesota Medicine*: Antibiotics, Por Favor (November 2007), Caring for Lucy (March 2009), Shining Light in Dark Places (August 2009), Reflections on an Untimely Death (April 2010), Field Clinics (September 2010) and The Medical Deity is Dead (December 2011). On the Navajo Reservations won the annual writing *Minnesota Medicine* prize in 2009 and was published in July 2009.

Lies, White Lies and the Truth was published as My Work: Discerning Lies, White Lies and the Truth in the anthology *MOTIF 3: Work*, Motes Books, 2011.

The Pilgrim's Journey was published in *Tiferet: A Spiritual Journal* in February 2011.

An early version of Second Guessing the Second Opinion and Meeting Daniel were published in *Archives of Pediatric and Adolescent*

Medicine, December 2004, Vol 158 and August 2005, Vol 159, respectively.

Dog Pals was originally published in JAMA, April 2006, Vol 259 and republished in Minnesota Medicine, April 2007.

An earlier version Reborn in Honduras was published *Family Medicine* in February 2005.

Thanks to the patients, colleagues and family who inspired the stories. Thanks to all who helped to shape my work. Writing mentors: Cynthia Bend and Catherine Friend. Editors: Cindy Rogers, Elizabeth Greene and Gary Gilmer. Fellow writers: Kay, Nancy, Bernie, Betty, Kathy, Maggie and those I've forgotten. Writing teachers: Mary Carroll Moore and Elizabeth Andrew at the Loft in Minneapolis, Minnesota (www.loft.org/), Mary Pierce Brosmer and teachers at Women Writing for (a) Change in Cincinnati, Ohio (www.womenwriting.org/).

My gratitude to the editors and publications who have appreciated and published my work over the years, especially Carmen Peota.

My heartfelt appreciation to Leslie Matton-Flynn, writing pal and graphic designer.

About The Author

Dr. Therese Zink is a family physician and professor at the University of Minnesota where she cares for patients, teaches and does research. She has written award-winning stories on doctoring. Her work has been published in both literary and medical journals as well as anthologies. She edited *The Country Doctor Revisited: A 21*st *Century Reader* (Kent State University, 2010), stories, poems and essays about rural health care today (www.thecountrydoctorrevisited.org) and *Becoming a Doctor: Reflections by Minnesota Medical Students* (Univeristy of Minnesota, 2011), a literary portrait of the many steps along the path to becoming a physician. Zink believes that reflection is an important ingredient for professionalism and staying grounded as a physician. She enjoys helping medical students write and publish the "interesting stories" that they post in on-line discussions or share during "significant event reflection" sessions while on their family medicine clerkships. She lives on twenty acres in southern Minnesota.